A Second Act

What Nearly Dying Teaches Us
About Really Living

Dr Matt Morgan

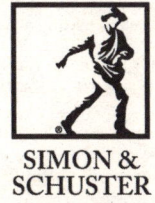

**SIMON &
SCHUSTER**

London · New York · Sydney · Toronto · New Delhi

First published in Great Britain by Simon & Schuster UK Ltd, 2025
This edition published in Great Britain by Simon & Schuster UK Ltd, 2026

Copyright © Dr Matt Morgan, 2025

The right of Dr Matt Morgan to be identified as the author of this work has been asserted in accordance with the Copyright, Designs and Patents Act, 1988.

1 3 5 7 9 10 8 6 4 2

Simon & Schuster UK Ltd, 1st Floor
222 Gray's Inn Road, London WC1X 8HB

For more than 100 years, Simon & Schuster has championed authors and the stories they create. By respecting the copyright of an author's intellectual property, you enable Simon & Schuster and the author to continue publishing exceptional books for years to come. We thank you for supporting the author's copyright by purchasing an authorised edition of this book.

No amount of this book may be reproduced or stored in any format, nor may it be uploaded to any website, database, language-learning model, or other repository, retrieval, or artificial intelligence system without express permission. All rights reserved. Enquiries may be directed to Simon & Schuster, 222 Gray's Inn Road, London WC1X 8HB or RightsMailbox@simonandschuster.co.uk

Simon & Schuster strongly believes in freedom of expression and stands against censorship in all its forms. For more information, visit BooksBelong.com.

www.simonandschuster.co.uk
www.simonandschuster.com.au
www.simonandschuster.co.in

Simon & Schuster Australia, Sydney
Simon & Schuster India, New Delhi

The authorised representative in the EEA is Simon & Schuster Netherlands BV, Herculesplein 96, 3584 AA Utrecht, Netherlands. info@simonandschuster.nl

Excerpt from 'Not Waving but Drowning' by Stevie Smith reprinted by permission of Faber and Faber Ltd.

The author and publishers have made all reasonable efforts to contact copyright-holders for permission, and apologise for any omissions or errors in the form of credits given. Corrections may be made to future printings.

A CIP catalogue record for this book is available from the British Library

While all clinical cases are based on real patients, some names and characteristics may have been changed to protect their privacy, some events compressed and some dialogue recreated.

Paperback ISBN: 978-1-3985-3236-6
eBook ISBN: 978-1-3985-3234-2

Typeset in Bembo Std by Palimpsest Book Production Ltd, Falkirk, Stirlingshire
Printed and Bound in the UK using 100% Renewable
Electricity at CPI Group (UK) Ltd

Dr Matt Morgan is a British intensive care doctor. His open letter addressed to patients during the 2020 Covid pandemic has been read by over half a million people worldwide and viewed over two million times after featuring on the Channel 4 news. His articles have featured in the *Guardian*, the *Telegraph*, the *Daily Mail*, the *Sunday Mirror* and the *Huffington Post*. A regular writer for the internationally acclaimed *British Medical Journal*, his article 'A letter from the ICU' is one of their most popular opinion articles, read by over 130,000 people in 2020. His first book, *Critical*, has been translated into four languages. He lives in Cardiff with his family, enjoys long walks with his dog, photography, cold beer and even colder ice cream.

Praise for *A Second Act*

'Combining vivid storytelling with thoughtful reflections ... *A Second Act* calls to something deep inside me, inside all of us, not to let the wonder of being alive pass us by. I hope this book reaches readers everywhere, to inspire and console them'
Dr Kathryn Mannix

'Morgan has a knack of writing simply and sincerely on matters that worry most of us ... dramatic and heart-warming'
The Times

'*A Second Act* has a neat narrative structure and covers a resonant subject, and Morgan is a thoughtful and sensitive writer ... [it] contains a lot of wisdom'
New Statesman

'Morgan proves an excellent guide to such wisdom. He is grateful to bear witness to these stories – and self-effacing about the part he plays in enabling some of them'
Observer

'Humbling and very moving. Absolutely essential reading for any healthcare professional'
Dr Xand van Tulleken

Also by Matt Morgan

Critical
One Medicine

To all the patients who didn't get to live their second act

Contents

Prologue: Aunty Win 1

1 Struck by Lightning 11
2 Blue Blood 26
3 Red Dust 59
4 Summer 74
5 Drowning not Waving 94
6 A Heart in a Jar 112
7 Go Nuts 131
8 3 Billion Beats 151
9 Heartless 183
10 Frozen Solid 209
11 A Funeral for my Friends 225

Epilogue 252
Acknowledgements 259

'There is only a moment between the past & the future. That moment we call life.'

Terry Pratchett

Prologue: Aunty Win

Win, ninety-seven years old
Cause of death: Life

I have some bad news – you are going to die. I am going to die. We are all going to die. Steve Jobs said, 'Death is life's greatest invention.' Eternal life would be no life at all. But what if there are people who have seen both sides? People who have glimpsed the darkness before returning to a new life? People in a rare 6 per cent club that survive intact after a cardiac arrest where their heart stops but starts again.* What might they be able to teach us? Life is lived forwards but best understood backwards, so let us begin not at the beginning but at the end.

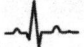

---

* This percentage differs according to country, which data is used and how 'intact' is defined. I'm using the latest statistics from Steven C. Brooks, Gareth R. Clegg, Janet Bray, Charles D. Deakin, Gavin D. Perkins, Mattias Ringh, Christopher M. Smith, et al,

I had never been to a funeral on my birthday. It wouldn't be the last time. In the years that followed Aunty Win's death, my life would change, stretch, warp and morph. I would become lost and then found thanks to lessons from the near dead that I have gathered together in this book. And then I would go to a second funeral on my birthday five years later that would help me live a better life.

Aunty Win died when she was ninety-seven. She had lived an extraordinary life and so didn't need her funeral to be sad. In many ways it wasn't. Yet, traditions and cultural norms frame them in sombre tones, emphasising loss over legacy. Her funeral was held under a sullen, pewter sky, as if nature itself was a mourner. Heavy wool coats and dark scarves wrapped thick around solemn necks. Leafless trees were silent witnesses, their skeletal branches reaching skyward. The crunch of frostbitten grass beneath my polished shoes was like a beat to move to as, with five others, I carried Win on my shoulder. The stone-hewn church offered refuge from the cold, damp earth mingling with a faint aroma of incense. As the casket was lowered, a gentle rain began to fall. The final farewells were whispered on the wind, carrying both sorrow and a poignant reminder of life's fragile beauty. I read out her

---

★ 'Optimizing Outcomes After Out-of-Hospital Cardiac Arrest With Innovative Approaches to Public-Access Defibrillation: A Scientific Statement From the International Liaison Committee on Resuscitation', Circulation, 2022, vol. 145, no. 13, e776–801, https://doi.org/10.1161/CIR.0000000000001013

Prologue: Aunty Win

eulogy in the form of a letter to break the sadness that tradition demanded:

Dear Aunty Win,
I've never written to someone who has died before. But it just seems apt. I wanted to write about you but then thought why not write to you? So, this is a letter not from me, but from us all here today, to say thanks, and hello and goodbye.

Ninety-seven years seems like a really long time: 5,044 Saturdays and lazy Sundays, 1,164 bright full Moons, six dark solar eclipses, seven houses, five jobs, two proposals. Three billion heartbeats.

But your story isn't just about how long, it's also about what you have seen, and heard, and said and lived:

The BBC being created, women over twenty-one getting the vote, penicillin being discovered, a king dying, a king abdicating, a new king, a new queen, the war, the Blitz, Churchill, D-Day, VE Day, the birth of the NHS, the Olympics in London, DNA being discovered, England winning the World Cup, the Beatles, Concorde, no more shillings, joining the EU, leaving the EU, the internet, mobile phones, presidents, prime ministers, film and music stars coming and going, but you stay.

But your story isn't just about how long you were here, or what you have seen, and heard, and said and lived. It's also about who you were, who you are, to us all then and now.

Daughter

Sister

Niece

Aunty

Farmhand

Like a mum to some

A rock

A confidante

A churchyard visitor

A source of pride, wisdom and inspiration

A dancer, a secretary, a war-time hero

A plotter of maps

A writer of a hundred cards every Christmas

A friend to so many

An endless supplier of biscuits and KitKats.

But Aunty Win to me

And loved by us all – now, yesterday and tomorrow,

Yours sincerely,

Friends, family and those lucky enough to have met you.

P.S.

Write back if you can.

It helped I think. As the final organ note ended, there was a palpable shift from solemnity to camaraderie. Mourners moved from the graveside to Win's house. The warmth and

Prologue: Aunty Win

solace came from each other's company. The atmosphere lightened; a hum of conversation mingled with the clinking of teacups; the damp church air replaced by freshly baked scones and wine.

A photo of Win on the table, a moment of joy frozen from a long, happy life. People gather around, pointing and reminiscing, their voices tinged with fondness and nostalgia. Win's favourite Welsh hymns looped in the background. Children play quietly in corners. Stories and laughter weave through the air like an invisible thread, connecting everyone, reaching out to Aunty Win. Then hugs and handshakes are exchanged, each gesture a silent pact to keep the memory of the departed alive. 'We must meet again soon.' They promise, knowing that the next time may be at their own funeral.

The gathering winds down, a sense of closure settles in. The mourners disperse, carrying with them the comforting reminder that life, in all its beauty and fragility, is best honoured by cherishing those who remain. It had been a lovely day. And then it struck me – Win would have loved this: the music, the people, the food, the readings. Win would have loved to be at her own funeral.

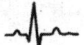

I've worked as an intensive care doctor for more than twenty years, caring for patients who are in thick fog, tiptoeing between life and death.

Intensive care doctor:
intensivist, critical care doctor, intensive care medicine doctor, resuscitationist. Ultimately, just a human going to work.

Although one in five of you admitted will eventually die in an intensive care unit, many of you won't even know what that is. The intensive care unit (ICU) is a place where the extraordinary becomes routine, a place where life hangs in a delicate balance, and every moment is a battle against the odds. It is also very ordinary – staff coming to work, tea being drunk, lunch breaks, printers jamming, toilets leaking. It is almost more surprising to me that astonishing things happen there thanks to very normal people and things. ICU is a microcosm of life, accelerated.

ICU didn't really exist in the 1940s when my dad was born. It was thanks to a global viral pandemic of polio in 1952 that a doctor called Dr Bjørn Ibsen inserted a pipe into the neck of a 12-year-old girl called Vivi, which laid the foundations for the modern ICU. But as ever, it isn't the procedures, machines or drugs that make an ICU great – it's the people working there. Vivi survived thanks to the teams of 1,500 medical students who squeezed a bag attached to the pipe in her neck for hours, then days, then weeks and months. She left hospital, thrived, fell in love and travelled thanks to people. And it was thanks to another global viral pandemic nearly seventy years later that those people who work in ICU were finally recognised in the *Oxford English Dictionary* as 'intensivists' – apparently I am 'a medical practitioner specialising in intensive care'. Ultimately, just a human going to work in an amazing place with a great group of people.

If you walk into ICU, the first thing you will notice is the symphony of beeps and hums from sophisticated machinery – ventilators, medication pumps, dialysis machines and monitors – all orchestrating to keep patients alive. Each bed is not at all a place of rest but a hub of activity, surrounded by state-of-the-art equipment and, most importantly, a dedicated nurse. These nurses, the unsung heroes of the ICU, provide round-the-clock care, ensuring that every heartbeat, every breath, is meticulously monitored.

The patients in ICU are the sickest in the hospital, battling severe organ failures – lungs that refuse to breathe, hearts that falter, kidneys that cease to filter. Their conditions are varied – severe infections, post-surgical complications, traumatic injuries, bodies that are attacking themselves. It is no wonder that I often feel unsure of myself when expected to instantly recall the 13,000 diagnoses, 6,000 drugs and 4,000 surgical procedures that are possible. I try to balance the logical science side of ICU with the humanity needed. I try not to think with my gut or shit with my brain.

The ICU is also a crucible of innovation. Inspired by practices from aviation and cognitive science, it has adopted checklists and crew resource management techniques to minimise errors and enhance patient safety. These strategies ensure that, despite the chaos, every patient receives the highest standard of care, tailored meticulously to their needs.

It does come at a price. A single night spent in intensive care can cost as much as £3,000. But it works. ICU saves lives. The average mortality rate for critically ill patients has been falling over time thanks to better systems, better training, better equipment and evidence-based therapies. There are now more than 30 million patients admitted to intensive care worldwide every year, of whom 24 million will survive. We can therefore estimate that, since that first patient, around half a billion people have survived thanks to ICU.

But beyond costs, technology and procedures, it is the more important emotional and ethical dimensions in life that lie at the heart of every ICU. This is a place where human resilience and fragility coexist, where every victory is hard-won, and every loss is deeply felt. The staff, constantly navigating a permacrisis, exhibit remarkable resilience, empathy and moral fortitude, supporting patients and their families through some of the darkest moments. But we are not only there to save a life. We also need to save a death. We play our part in the four out of five people who survive ICU, but we also need to care for the one out of five who sadly do not.

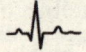

Prologue: Aunty Win

I've met hundreds of people whose hearts have stopped – they died and then they were resuscitated and lived. In the long days and short years that followed Aunty Win's funeral, I began to realise that compared with business gurus or social media influencers, it is these patients who survive their unscheduled meeting with death who are the people we really should be listening to. They know what really matters.

And so, after Win's funeral, I started collecting the words spoken by these patients, their thoughts and their answers to tricky questions. In a small red book that I always kept on me at work, I scrawled down what I call their 'whispers of life'. We've all heard these lessons before – in poetry, in song lyrics and spoken by people we love. But only after touching death and being confronted by our own mortality can we really turn up the volume on these whispers. Only then can they be heard clearly. Because life is best understood backwards but lived forwards. And with one in 100 people dying every year,* what better time to listen to these whispers than now? When you are in the ninety-nine out of 100 still alive.

I want to tell you about these lessons from the patients I have cared for. Each died in a different way – two friends hit by lightning, a woman with no heart, a fisherman who slept with the fishes, a man buried by snow and a doctor

---

* According to the CIA's *The World Factbook*, this varies from as many as nineteen deaths per 1,000 population each year in Ukraine to just one per 1,000 population per year in Qatar.

with a broken heart. We will meet them in their first life, witness their death and understand how they were resuscitated, before returning to meet them in their second act. We will see how they changed and what lessons we can all learn to better enjoy our own time on this small blue dot. Because if funerals are wasted on the dead, then life is wasted on the living.

1

STRUCK BY LIGHTNING

Ed, forty-seven years old
Cause of death: Lightning
Cause of life: Talk about love, talk about the dead

Ed remembers the day he died. Being a 17-year-old, football-mad teenager growing up in a small English town, Friday night meant one thing – the pub with friends. Speaking with Ed three decades later, now forty-seven, he carries the weight of years marked by life's fiercest storms, emerging scarred yet resilient. He wore a blue zip-up hoodie, the bright white zipper matching the speckles of white in his well-groomed beard, the straight line of white up his chest like the lightning bolt that hit Ed and his best friend Stuart three decades ago. Ed got a second act, but Stuart did not.

Ed was born in the small town of Kenilworth in Warwickshire, England. His dad was a hard-working, no-nonsense chartered electrical engineer, while his mum stayed at home to care for Ed and his two brothers. After moving around the country for his dad's work, the family returned to their home town when Ed was ten. His brothers started university, leaving Ed effectively an only child, but he had plenty to keep him busy. Good school grades didn't come easily, partly as a result of Ed studying subjects his parents wanted him to rather than following his more creative passions. But school wasn't just for grades, it was also for friends, who made Ed's life a lot of fun.

He told me about the reassuring rhythms to small town life – hanging out in the park after school, then Thursday would be for planning Friday night and Friday night for planning Saturday night. Smoky pubs where everyone knew (and had kissed) everyone. It reminded me of my own teenage years in a gritty Welsh town called Neath, where, by coincidence, Ed's godmother lived. For teenaged Ed, every weekend was the same, apart from one every June. And in June 1994 it was terribly different.

On the last weekend of June, the fair came to Kenilworth. There were rides, a carnival, overpriced and undercooked hot dogs for sale, as well as kitchen gadgets that you buy but never use. Nestled in the picturesque grassland of Abbey Fields, the fair was surrounded by hills used for sledging in the winter.

After an early trip to the pub, Ed and his four friends ventured to the fair. As the sun started to dip, the group walked home across the fields towards the main road. Ed's best friend Stuart needed to get a taxi home because his parents were away on holiday in Europe. At sixteen, Stuart was the youngest of the group, and his small yet stocky frame suited his fly-half position in the nearby Leamington rugby team. He and Ed had become close after Stuart joined the local sixth-form college. They would often have a milky instant coffee together at Ed's house before Stuart's cycle ride home.

As the fairground noises faded behind the group, the rain started. Heavy rain, quickly soaking the jumpers they held above their heads. Stuart and his girlfriend sheltered under one of the large oak trees that dotted the field while Ed walked ahead with his friend Emma.

"And then, *bang!*" Ed described, holding up his hands, palms facing me.

That bang was a powerful bolt of forked lightning – 300 million volts; enough energy to power my home city of Cardiff for a whole day. Emma flew backwards, arms and legs stretched out like in a star jump. Ed remembers a glow and then being violently pulled downwards towards the ground. 'I felt like a can being crushed,' he told me. And then he died.

The cause of a cardiac arrest from a lightning strike is often direct damage to the heart cells that control the heartbeat. One short circuit can cut the connections needed to keep the heart beating in time, a fault not dissimilar to those Ed's dad encountered in his work across the telephone networks of Europe. Lightning can also cause severe burns, both on the body's surface and inside the organs, as well as kidney failure from the resulting muscle breakdown. And while there are treatments that can be given, you first must arrive at the hospital – alive. Restarting the heart using CPR as quickly as possible to reduce any brain damage is key. The longer the delay, the more the brain is starved of blood. And your brain is a hungry organ, needing three times the amount of oxygen-rich blood compared with your heart muscle. Without this constant feast, millions of nerve cells, tiny pieces of wire wrapped in fat, die every second. In other words, during a cardiac arrest, time is brain and brain is you.

The noise from the lightning strike was so loud it was heard at the fire station 200 metres away. One of the volunteer firemen, who'd been about to get in his car to go home, ran through the rain towards the scene, not knowing what he would find. The body he saw first was Ed's. As he did CPR, he saw another under the oak tree. That was Stuart. Because Ed was found first, he lived. For Stuart, it was sadly too late.

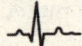

Think of all the plans you have ever made, the lists of pros and cons to help you make a decision, sleepless nights wrestling over option A or B. Should you end a relationship or take a new job? Move overseas or stay at home? We feel that we control our lives. We act like we are the arbitrators. But this is an illusion.

Most of the major forks in life's road happen due to pure chance. To start at the beginning, you were born, despite the chances of this being infinitesimally small. Then you managed not to die as a baby or child. You didn't choose the genes that made you brave or strong or motivated or lazy. You probably fell in love with someone you could easily have never come across, whether you met at an airport, at school, at work or thanks to an algorithm. Every event in your life, no matter how seemingly insignificant, has led you through a million doors to allow you to read these words on the page here and now. That is wild. Sometimes I think we are made out of luck.

Why Ed lived and Stuart died was down to pure chance. A portion of good and a measure of bad. Had Ed been the one sitting at the base of the tree, I would have been speaking with Stuart instead. If that fireman had clocked off early, or was sick, or the station was a mile further away, both boys would have died. Lady luck isn't always ladylike. As it happened, Ed received CPR within minutes of his heart stopping, and got to live. Stuart received CPR moments later and would die.

Luck runs both ways. Every day, I care for patients who are critically ill in the Intensive Care Unit, some because of bad luck, and some because of bad choices. They have drunk too much, driven too fast, done something stupid. Yet I too have drunk too much, driven too fast and done stupid things. I was lucky. They were unlucky. They will die or go to jail, and I will not.

The Oxford philosopher Derek Parfit calls this 'moral luck'. He describes situations where the moral judgement of someone's actions depends on factors beyond their control. Parfit highlights how the ethical evaluation of actions varies depending on their outcomes, many of which are influenced by chance. Two drivers might act equally negligently, but only one hits a pedestrian who ends up in my ICU. And the reason for this difference is not the degree of negligence, but rather circumstances beyond their control: bad luck. Society and the law judge the driver involved in the accident more harshly, even though both drivers exhibited the same level of carelessness. This hardly seems fair. Recognising the influence of uncontrollable factors, we can approach others with greater compassion and understanding, acknowledging the complex factors that shape our moral landscape.

It can allow us to see people not only as their worst mistake. People are not a single thing, not only the result of their worst moral luck. And knowing how much of our lives are dictated by chance gives us that gap between stimulus and response to not be smug about our success nor bitter about our losses. The time to make up your mind about someone is never. If there is a god, he does play dice.

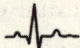

As the firefighter pressed down on Ed's chest, squeezing blood to his brain, Ed woke up.

'We've got him!' said someone in the crowd that had gathered from the nearby fair. Strangers picked up Ed and ran him down the hill underneath an umbrella. The streetlights had turned a strange colour and Ed remembers feeling like he was being carried on a rubber ring surrounded by soft flowing currents of light. Then his heart stopped again.

'We've lost him!'

After another round of CPR, Ed woke up in the ambulance that then took him to the cardiac unit at nearby Warwick hospital. In the early hours of the morning, he was unable to sleep, and a well-intentioned nurse asked him, 'Have you ever lost a friend before?' Walking down the corridor, Ed saw one of Stuart's brothers crying, waiting for his parents to return from Europe. Stuart had died from the lack of blood supply to his brain, just one week before his seventeenth birthday.

In many ways, Ed was the norm, Stuart just very unlucky. Nine out of ten people struck by lightning survive. That's because direct strikes make up only a tiny portion of all lightning strikes. Instead, most injuries happen when lightning travels through the ground from some distance away. Ed had simply been further away than Stuart from the point of impact. He may have even been hit just by a side flash, when current jumps between an object like a tree and the person, causing what is known as 'flashover'. These two types of indirect strikes are far more likely and far less deadly than a direct lightning strike.

But when a bolt does pass straight through the body, the heart often stops and then only CPR will help. The quicker the better, with every minute of delay decreasing the chances of survival by 10 per cent. Stuart had been unlucky to be hit directly, Ed lucky to have received CPR so quickly.

Ed was released from hospital the next day. Emma, who had been sent flying through the air, had needed only minor treatment at the scene. Stuart's girlfriend was uninjured. Ed's hospital property bag included a drawing made in those sleepless hours, of his own body lying on the ground, seen from above. The metal buttons on Ed's denim jacket were drawn warped, his belt buckle twisted and burned. His parents later showed him the jacket with the same warped buttons and the twisted, burned belt buckle.

There were reporters waiting outside his house as the police interviewed Ed. It was the first time he had seen raw emotion from his dad, who sat shaking, wanting to hold Ed's hand during the police's questioning, but not knowing if he could or should.

Walking around his home town, Ed always felt eyes on him. He was the lightning guy. The one that died and yet was saved. The lucky one. We all make exaggerated caricatures of those close to us. Friendship groups or families have the quiet one, the crazy one, the one who dances, the one who always puts their foot in it. Ed had been distilled down to one thing. Not even the pub was the same. There were whispers and laughs and glances. A spotlight followed him everywhere he went. He would later move away to Leeds to try to find some shade, but instead landed in the shadow of drugs and alcohol.

The psychological 'spotlight effect' describes a human tendency to overestimate the attention others pay to our appearance, actions or mistakes. Like Ed, many of us can feel like we are on stage with a spotlight pointed directly at us. In reality, people are seldom as focused on us as we think. Many people do not care about you – and that can be a good thing.

In the classic experiment demonstrating this spotlight effect, participants donned a T-shirt with a large, embarrassing image of Barry Manilow before walking into a packed room. They were then asked to estimate the number of people in the room who noticed the T-shirt they were wearing. Most greatly overestimated the number who had noticed the shirt, guessing it was over 50 per cent. The true number was less than 20 per cent.

In everyday life, this human tendency can lead to unnecessary stress and anxiety. In medical school, I remember falling sideways out of my seat during a particularly boring lecture. I hadn't fallen asleep but instead was reaching forwards to pick up my pen from the floor. I tumbled twenty rows down the stairs from the top to the bottom of the large lecture theatre. I landed on my back, looking upwards at a rather angry yet bemused lecturer. I was mortified, although as I learned in the coffee break, many of my friends hadn't even noticed this theatrical stunt.

Understanding the spotlight effect can be liberating. It encourages us to be more forgiving of ourselves, recognising that others are less judgemental and observant of our flaws than we fear. By dimming the imagined spotlight, we can navigate social situations with greater ease and confidence, focusing less on perceived judgements and more on genuine interaction and self-expression. This awareness can lead to a healthier self-image and more authentic connections with others, as we realise that everyone is the main character in their own story, not a spectator in ours.

It can be powerful to know that no one really cares. But there are times when you need someone to care, you need a spotlight to show you the way, or to at least give some warmth as a side effect of the light.

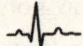

In the days that followed Stuart's death, Ed's second act was spent sitting in his bedroom with the curtains closed. People came round but he didn't want to see them. Soon came Stuart's funeral, and Ed found the strength somewhere to do a reading. The school had organised a bus to the service from a school trip the children were on in Durham. It had been the first time that Ed had left the house but being surrounded by friends again slowly pulled back the curtains on his grief.

Ed simply didn't know how to process what had happened. And people didn't ask him about it either. Worried about saying the wrong thing, most people said nothing. Yet nothing is always the wrong thing to say. Ed spent years living with what he now recognises as survivor guilt. He made many bad life choices in the years that followed, trying to answer questions like, 'Why me?' 'Why him?' 'Why us?'

It's hard enough being seventeen and navigating life, let alone when you carry the death of your best friend everywhere you go. Ed didn't return to the fair the next June or the June after that. He either loved or hated thunderstorms depending on his mood. Sometimes Ed avoided Abbey Fields and took a much longer route home. Sometimes he would go there on purpose and sit under that oak tree by himself for hours. Ed no longer feared death at all. He didn't care if he woke up the next day or not. He was never suicidal and enjoyed the life he led at that moment. But the consequences of his actions weren't what he cared about. He didn't feel he deserved to be alive, so there was little to lose. What he did lose were hours and days of his life at a time, consumed by the metal music club scene and the alcohol or drugs that for him became an integral part of it.

Today, losing the fear of death is something many strive for. The psychedelic revolution of the '70s was marginalised through the actions of people like Timothy Leary, who famously said, 'Tune in, drop out.' Fifty years later, psychedelics are back on the prescription pad for people with terminal diseases who want to get to that place where Ed lost his fear of death. Dying certainly seems to help reduce anxiety related to the end of life.

In my last book, *One Medicine*, we met Chris Lemons, a deep-sea saturation diver who died for forty-five minutes when his oxygen supply was disconnected. He lay fitting on the ocean floor yet lived to tell the tale. After being rescued, Chris said about death: 'You do know it's okay, don't you? It's just like drifting off to sleep. I was sad for a bit. I was cold and got a bit numb but then it was just like falling asleep. It's not that bad.' In fact, staying very cold can be a superpower.

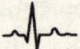

Unfortunately, unlike Chris Lemons brushing off death, it didn't feel like that for Ed. Although he no longer feared his own death, Ed continued to struggle after losing those around him. Over the next year, three people close to Ed died. One in a car crash, a friend who died by suicide, and Ed's grandad. Yet Ed remained alone in his grief. There were no support services apart from an annual check on his heart. It was broken, but not medically.

I asked Ed if he would say anything to that 17-year-old boy now, thirty years later.

'Yeah, loads,' he said, nodding his head slowly. 'I would say, "You are not alone". I would throw my arms around him. I would say that this will pass.'

Thankfully, healthcare has realised that simply fixing bodies and bones is not enough. The heart checks that Ed went for at his local hospital were all fine, but what he needed was someone to listen, to hold him. To ask the difficult questions:

'How are you managing with the death of your best friend?'

'Do you want to talk about it?'

'Tell me about Stuart. What was he like?'

'What do you miss about him?'

We are getting better at this kind of support, but it's still not good enough. Although support is in place for many patients and the families of patients with chronic diseases including cancer, this isn't the case when it comes to sudden bereavement. Even in the intensive care unit, where death is a familiar face, with as many as one in five people dying, death sometimes feels like an afterthought, an add on. We should really be incredible at managing death and supporting those affected. We should be as good as we are at putting plastic tubes into lungs and restarting hearts. Yet bereavement support is often difficult to access. I am very proud to be an ambassador for the charity 2Wish, who aim to close this divide for those who have lost someone under the age of twenty-five. They provide support in those hours, days and weeks that really matter. But it is still a charity. Is universal healthcare universal if it stops at death?

Ed unknowingly created his own cure. All bad choices have a story behind them, and Warwick hospital understood this. They accepted Ed to work as a volunteer in the years after Stuart's death. During quiet times, Ed would walk the same corridors stained by Stuart's brother's tears, talking with people who were going through tough times. He then moved to social services, supporting children whose parents were unwell with cancer. He gave the help, the time and the questions that he himself had wanted. He knew that sometimes the best things to offer are not answers but just your presence, even when you have nothing to say.

So, if this is you, if you know someone struggling and can't think of the right thing to say, just say something. Or say nothing but be there. Tell them you love them. Tell them you care. Tell them you are there. Do it now. Because you may not get a second chance.

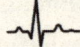

Ed and I had been speaking for hours. As evening fell, the white zipper on his hoodie seemed a little less bright than before. His story is stunning not because of the lightning. It is amazing because of what that lightning hit. Because of the people.

'I still live with it every day,' Ed said. 'But now I am living with it, not reliving it.'

'If you could press a button that would have stopped this ever happening, would you?' I asked.

He took a while to answer, changing his position in his seat a few times.

'I would press it for Stuart, of course, and for that 17-year-old. But not for this 47-year-old. Because I am here because of it. And because of my son Toby. I didn't know if I really wanted kids. But me and my son Toby have been a team since he was three. Just the two of us. We are a great team. He's the best thing that happened in my life.'

Toby has just turned fourteen. He too goes to Kenilworth School. The weekend before Ed and I spoke, Toby had marched in the remembrance parade across Abbey Fields, past that oak tree. The fireman who saved Ed was marching alongside him.

Perhaps Ed sees Stuart when he looks at his son.

'I had never thought of that,' he said. 'But I tell him I love him every day. I say how proud he makes me. And how I'll always be there no matter what. And I would say the same things to Stuart.'

2

BLUE BLOOD

Luca, thirty years old
Cause of death: Covid
Cause of life: Words have power

We have two lives. The second begins when you realise you have one. For Luca, a 30-year-old Italian pharmacist living in Wales, this realisation came in 2020 when he died from Covid.

Luca grew up in an apartment tucked away in southern Rome. His mum was a teacher and his dad a banker, born the same year as intensive care was invented. Luca's childhood was spent hanging out with friends, going to the cinema and being teased for not following the national religion of football. He loved science as a kid, although regularly missed school with a stream of childhood illnesses. What his friends would brush off as a minor cough or cold would make Luca seriously unwell and take him much longer to recover. It was his frustration with ill health that led Luca to qualify as a pharmacist.

Although he loved his job, even before his brush with death, Luca knew there was more to life than just his own beautiful but familiar city. By 2011, he had booked airline tickets to swap his Apennine mountains of Italy for the green hills of Wales. His bags lay packed on his bedroom floor when a chance encounter at a party led him to meet his future partner, Aria. Luca soon realised he would be leaving behind someone very special but, given the many plans that were already in place, the new couple exchanged Skype usernames and left their future to chance, kissing goodbye after one final trip to Venice.

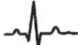

In life, timing is as crucial as the choices we make. Understanding this explains why Luca was right to fly away. This is vividly illustrated by the viral image of an elderly couple sleeping in a gondola on Venice's Grand Canal, where Luca and Aria spent their last day together. The photo shows a couple in their seventies sprawled over each other, both fast asleep with the gondolier smiling in amusement to himself. Perhaps they had dreamed of visiting Venice for decades, saving enough until the time was just right, the bank balance enough, the kids settled. When that day came, they found themselves too tired and too old to fully enjoy it. Their peaceful slumber during a once-in-a-lifetime experience serves as a visual reminder of the importance of seizing the right time.

The book *Four Thousand Weeks*, by the self-confessed

productivity junkie Oliver Burkeman, reminds us that our time on Earth is limited – averaging around 4,000 weeks, just 28,000 days. This finite span means prioritisation is key, making sure what truly matters is grasped when the timing is right. Waiting for that 'perfect' moment often results in missed opportunities. Yes, Luca could have delayed his move abroad, but would this change ever be possible again?

Instead, the right time is often now, rather than in some distant, uncertain future. Or at least, there are activities where the time must be now to fully embrace them. Starting a family, pursuing a dream job, travelling to new places. Each requires not just the right choice but also the right timing. Delaying these decisions can mean losing out on the experiences and growth they offer. And being sad after making a decision doesn't mean it was the wrong decision.

In essence, timing and choice are intertwined threads in the fabric of a well-lived life. And certain things are best done at predictable, specific times in life. Bill Perkins, in *Die with Zero*, argues that the greatest fulfilment comes from experiences that match the right timing of our lives. Ski when you are young even if you can't afford it because when you are rich and seventy, your knees will not forgive you. Take adventurous trips in youth, invest in relationships throughout your middle years and savour reflective moments in older age. This approach ensures we extract the most value and joy from our life's timeline, aligning our actions with our stage of life.

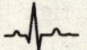

Two years after leaving Aria in Italy, after countless phone calls, video messages, flights to meet for birthdays and holidays, Luca proposed in Sardinia. They married in Rome during summer 2016, and after a tough pregnancy, their beautiful daughter, Sofia, was born in May 2019. Just a year after Luca's life was turned upside down by becoming a dad, another tiny life-form would do it once again.

Luca had been working overtime as a hospital pharmacist during April 2020, handing out medicines to help patients with Covid. On a rare day off, pushing his daughter's pram along the River Taff close to his house felt unusually difficult. After getting home, Luca's skin started heating up. His temperature climbed higher at night and soon came a dry, annoying cough. Struggling on for the next few days, he took his own professional advice by drinking plenty of water, taking paracetamol to help his temperature and the banging headache. But as the next Sunday came around, Luca's temperature hit 40 degrees, his cough stopped him sleeping and his breathing sounded like an old church organ.

Luca drove himself to my hospital, passing his pharmacy colleagues in the corridors as his bed was quickly pushed to a Covid ward because his breathing was so fast. By midnight Luca's oxygen levels plummeted to levels lower than in climbers at the top of Mount Everest. He needed to go to the Intensive Care Unit for extra oxygen to be pushed under pressure into his lungs.

'I was actually relieved to go to intensive care,' he told

me. 'I rang Aria and said not to worry, everything would be okay.'

An hour later, Luca was tired, the extra oxygen still wasn't enough. Not wanting to wake her, he sent Aria a text message saying he was going to be put on to a life support machine. The message ended simply with 'I love you x.' Then he sent a message to his boss: 'I won't be in work tomorrow.'

That night, I also rang Aria. Everything was not okay.

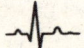

Intensive care doesn't really have outpatient clinics or waiting lists. If a patient needs to wait even an hour for life-saving treatment, then that is too long. And so I seldom write letters that are posted to GPs or sent to the patient's home. Instead, most of the words I use are written directly in hospital notes. These entries used to take a formulaic, structured style, full of bullet points, lists and strange symbols. Even if my doctor's handwriting was neat (which it is not), my notes would still look more like hieroglyphs than English, incomprehensible to patients themselves. But the pandemic changed that.

The whole world wanted to make sense of the story that was unfolding. And so my notes changed from reading like an academic textbook to like the pages of a book found on a coffee shop's table. I wasn't trying to pen a thriller or crime drama, but a biography of the patient I was caring for, weaving the science with the human, the worry with the hope. I wanted to make my notes understandable to all, not knowing who may read them in the future. After all, medicine should and must be a humane science, a scientific expression of the human condition. My long lists and strange symbols morphed into narrative, a tightly constructed paragraph to explain to other doctors, to me, and to the families of those who couldn't be there, what was going on. Using bullet points did allow me to take aim at diseases, but they would often miss the heart of the matter. So now I tried to make sense of each story through words. I still wrote prescriptions to heal bodies but now narratives to heal minds.

After I made this change, something else seemed odd. We try as doctors to put patients at the centre of all that we do. Yet the perpetual record of clinical encounters excludes patients from their own story. Medical notes are addressed to other doctors, written about patients. Not to them. After speaking with Luca's wife that night, I did something I had never done before. I'm not sure why or if I even thought about it. Despite Luca being unconscious and dying, I addressed my notes to him, like I was writing a letter just as I had done to my Aunty Win for her funeral. I desperately hoped this wouldn't be a eulogy.

> Hi Luca, I had a long chat with your wife, Aria, by phone tonight and could hear your young daughter, Sofia, in the background. I explained that you were critically unwell, needing all the oxygen that we could

give you through our life support machines. We have turned you to lie on your front, but this is not helping. I told Aria that you are sick enough to die. I'm very sorry that hearing this made her cry, but I wanted to be honest.

But there is hope. We wouldn't keep you alive like this if there was not. The reason I come to work every day is to get people like you back to the people who love them, like your wife and your daughter, Sofia. I said to Aria that I've asked a specialist team in London for one final treatment called ECMO. This could add oxygen directly to your blood, bypassing your lungs, which are full of fluid and infection. It might not work, and if it doesn't, you will die. But there is hope. It might work. And then you might live.

Words have power. Reading and writing have long affected me deeply. They seem to bypass an emotional electric fence that keeps me strong when talking to relatives or speaking to large audiences on stage. I also often write what is difficult to say and read what is difficult for me to hear to sneak through a gap in my own emotional perimeter. After I wrote these words to Luca, there was something extra left on the page in front of me, a tear from my own eye.

It is easier to find tears in hospital than water to drink. But collecting them all together still wouldn't cry enough for a river. It would need everyone on Earth to cry at least fifty tears to fill the equivalent 2.5 million litres of an Olympic swimming pool.

Only humans cry because of emotions. Tears can spring forth from the simplest stimuli – a poignant memory, a piece of music or the joy of a reunion. They cleanse the eyes of irritants, but emotional tears serve a deeper, more mysterious purpose. They are the body's way of releasing stress, a silent language that speaks our inner turmoil or joy.

The act of crying is not just a release but also a form of communication. It signals distress, asks for empathy and support from those around us. Crying can strengthen bonds and foster community, ensuring that we are not alone in our moments of greatest vulnerability. This is why crying in response to emotional pain, such as grief or loss, can be profoundly therapeutic.

The theory that crying helps us deal with loss is supported by both psychological and physiological evidence. Emotional tears are known to contain higher levels of stress hormones like cortisol. By shedding these tears, we may be physically ridding our bodies of stress, leading to a calming effect. Psychologically, crying can act as a cathartic release, helping to process and accept grief. It allows us to confront and express our deepest emotions, facilitating a path towards healing.

Are we the only animals that cry? The short answer is no, but with caveats. Many animals produce tears for physiological reasons, like keeping their eyes moist or clearing debris. However, the phenomenon of crying in response to emotional stimuli seems uniquely human.

Human tears, therefore, remain one of our defining traits, a blend of the primal and the profoundly human. They are both a biological necessity and a profound statement of our emotional complexity. Through our tears, we connect, heal and express what words often cannot. That single tear I left on the page landed directly on the word hope. It blurred my blue ink but made it clearer than ever.

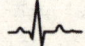

A few hours after my call for help, the team from London arrived. They drove on quiet streets, past closed shops and pubs as life had been put on pause by the government. Even the churches were closed on that Sunday. Perhaps this was the first time that organised religion had ever really listened to science.

But when they arrived, it wasn't as simple as just adding oxygen directly to Luca's blood. Luca first needed to be moved from his delicate position, tiptoeing on the shoreline between life and death in the ICU to the operating theatre. The machine that added oxygen needed thick plastic pipes to be inserted in blood vessels deep inside Luca's groin, fed along the inside of his body like an underground tunnel towards his heart. Plumbing these in safely needed millimetre precision, X-ray guidance and a sterile environment to prevent damaging his blood vessels, to stop Luca bleeding to death.

Even moving Luca was tough as Covid had shut down the theatres close to ICU. Instead, we needed to move him to a distant area normally used for replacing knees and hips. As well as being an intensive care doctor that day, I needed to be a locksmith and search for keys, an electrician to operate banks of light switches and a removal man to bring boxes of equipment. We needed to bring the operating theatre to life so that Luca could be brought back to life.

We delicately pushed Luca down the longest hospital corridor in Europe, still lying on his front attached to the countless leads and pipes of the life support machine. After arriving in the operating theatre, the whole team knew the next hour would mean the difference between life and death. Before any new pipes could be inserted, Luca needed to be returned to lying on his back. But simply doing this caused his oxygen levels to plummet even further. The monitor screamed out as Luca's blood oxygen saturations counted down from the mid-80s, a life threateningly low number, to the 70s then 60s. Numbers not compatible with life. Luca's heart struggled, slowed down to a stop. For a brief moment, life had gone, paused, his blue body looked already dead. I mentally prepared for the next conversation with Luca's wife, imagining her holding his daughter. I planned what words I would say. 'Died.' 'Painless.' 'Sorry.' Then I thought of my own daughter, Evie. It was her birthday. I had promised to be home on time. But it had already been hours since her candles had been blown out.

Then the complex machine that the London team had

brought started spinning. Pumps whirled, pipes rattled with the deep blue blood being sucked out from Luca's body, the colour of azure paint on a delicate porcelain vase, threading an intricate pattern through its surface-like veins in the body. The blue blood from Luca dived through the core of the machine in translucent pipes, ejected the other side like a fast-flowing river of bright red blood. This new blood was the intensity of a roaring fire, its warmth and energy coursing through Luca's veins like a relentless blaze.

This redness flowed into Luca's leg, up his body, turning his face from ashen to an ember glow. The monitor's screaming changed to a new ever rising tone, higher and higher, as his oxygen levels rose to the normal range for the first time in a week. The drugs we had been using to keep Luca alive were spooled down and within minutes all the pumps could be turned off completely. This was the moment between the past and the future. The moment we call life. It was like magic. The team prepared to transport Luca, still attached to their machine, to London.

Luca was the unlucky lucky one in those pandemic years. Many would never make it in time for this treatment and the team had to say 'no' far more than 'yes' to the phone calls for help coming in from all around the country. I remember Luca because he was rare, but I cannot forget the many patients, old and young, that didn't make it. Although many of us talk to the dead, they only spoke back to me in my dreams at night. In the years since, the dead have managed to stay with me, and even grow taller. Perhaps, or certainly, this was one reason why in the years that followed, I needed to change my own life.

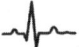

A year after I cared for Luca, a project was launched by my friend and colleague Jack Parry-Jones to plant a tree for each person we cared for during the pandemic. For the many that didn't make it, this paired remembrance and hope through new life. On a windy day, in a picturesque town nestling in the beautiful Usk Valley, my youngest daughter and I went to help plant these trees. For every patient cared for over the past year, and every staff member who worked tirelessly, a tree was planted. It was a poignant way to honour their memories and struggles, and it also provided a tangible connection to nature's healing power.

Jack was inspired to start this project by Viktor E. Frankl's book, *Man's Search for Meaning*. The Austrian neurologist, psychiatrist and Holocaust survivor was well-placed to argue we all need meaning in our lives. It was thanks to meaning that Frankl survived the horrors of his concentration camp. In Luca's case, meaning came from relationships with his wife and daughter. For others, purpose is found through work or spirituality and religion, perhaps personal growth or even their contribution to society. Others find worth in creativity and expression, experiences and adventure or even legacy. Jack realised that those who thrive after surviving critical care are those with meaning or hope in their lives.

In the wake of Covid, meaning and hope were thinning from people's lives and deaths. Jack approached the charity Stump Up For Trees as he felt planting trees might be a way to add meaning and commemorate patients and our staff as well as offset some of the carbon footprint from our critical care unit.

There now stands a woodland with 1,400 trees native to the Welsh hillside – hazel, wild cherry, blackthorn, sweet chestnut, oak and hawthorn. 'We need a world worth living in and biodiversity helps provide value to our lives.' Jack told me on that windswept day. The ICU is life on overdrive, a high-stakes blur of urgency and intensity. It is nice to think more slowly by immersing oneself in greenery, knowing the trees we planted will take decades not seconds to change. This experience was more than just an act of planting; it was a moving tribute to those we lost and a therapeutic process for those of us left behind.

Planting trees has long been associated with physical and mental health benefits. I met the wonderful James Wong, a British ethnobotanist who trained at London's Kew Gardens with both Welsh and Malaysian human roots. We were fellow panellists at the Hay Festival, a vibrant celebration of literature that transforms the town of Hay-on-Wye into a bustling hub of creativity and thought. Often dubbed 'the Woodstock of the mind', this ten-day event, beginning in late May, draws writers, thinkers and book lovers from all over the world.

James and I appeared together on a live BBC radio

comedy show where guests argued over what was the world's 'best medicine'. I claimed that animals were healthcare's most powerful treatment after writing my book *One Medicine*, which explored the profound connections between human and animal health. I was sure I would win, not least because I was armed with facts like the kangaroo has three vaginas and a whale's penis is actually called a 'pink floyd'.

James, however, swept in with a brilliant alternative, won over the crowd and took home the trophy. He showed how nature plays a crucial role in our emotional and physical well-being. Horticulture, he said, was clearly the best medicine. Being surrounded by greenery helps lower stress levels, reduce blood pressure and improve overall mood. This connection to nature is especially vital during times of crisis, like the pandemic, when many people turned to green spaces for solace and rejuvenation as we did in the forest. Perhaps the reason I was so happy that day at the Hay Festival was not because of the books that surrounded me, or the green room filled with my favourite literary celebrities, or even the overpriced ice cream. I was happy, James argued, because we were deep within the lush nature of mid-Wales, where the grass really is greener.

The human eye has even evolved to detect many more shades of green than any other colour. This evolutionary trait allowed our ancestors to distinguish between toxic and tasty plants, and now it enhances our appreciation of the natural world. James shared a fascinating study where participants on treadmills viewed different scenes while their stress levels were measured. Those who saw green environments found the exercise easier, felt better and had improved self-esteem compared to those who saw black and white or red-filtered views. This highlights how green spaces are somehow hardwired into positively affecting our perception and mood.

It is no wonder then that community gardens significantly combat loneliness and isolation, key factors in poor mental health. Engaging in gardening fosters social interactions, even for introverts. Of course, these benefits of horticulture are complex and individualised. What matters most is finding a personal connection to nature. Whether it's through a lush garden or a simple plant on a windowsill. Or for me and my daughter, planting trees to remember the lost from my past, to think about hope for the future and to plan the next birthday cake, which I hoped to make it home in time for.

So, although James won, my loss was worth me realising that our time making a new woodland was not just about planting trees. It was a therapeutic journey. The act of planting, feeling the soil, and working alongside others who shared our grief and hope was deeply healing. The trees we planted will stand as a testament to resilience and recovery, offering a peaceful spot for reflection for this lifetime and the next. As they grow over decades and generations, they will also contribute to a healthier environment, supporting local ecosystems and providing cleaner air. This initiative underscores the dual benefits of such projects: honouring those we've lost while promoting mental and environmental health.

Moreover, the initiative aligns with broader findings that urban greenery can significantly improve public health. Studies indicate that increased tree canopy cover in urban areas correlates with reduced stress, lower crime rates and better overall mental health. This project in Wales is a step towards creating a more sustainable and mentally supportive community. In the end, the windy day spent with my daughter planting trees was a day of connection – to nature, to each other and to the memories of those we lost. I found myself discussing difficult topics from those dark Covid days and nights with colleagues, made easier, less intimidating because I wasn't facing them. I couldn't see their eyes; they couldn't see mine. The movement and surroundings provided a comforting backdrop, making it easier to open up. It reminded us that from grief can come growth, and from loss, new life.

We wanted to give our woodland a name that would resonate deeply with its purpose and spirit. The decision to choose a name in Welsh was a tribute to our heritage and the local community. We believed that the right name could encapsulate the memory, peace and gratitude we wished to express through this woodland. After much deliberation, we narrowed our choices down to four names: Coed Cofio (Trees to Remember), Llecyn Llonydd (Peaceful Spot), Dail Diolch (Leaves of Thanks) and the eventual winner. A skilled local woodworker, Mick, battled through long Covid by carving a bench made from local beech and sweet chestnut. It sits proudly at the top of the site, overlooking the growing forest. I recently sat there, next to the plaque set deeply into its wooden layers translated into the many languages spoken by our diverse staff, including Spanish, Urdu, Polish and Portuguese. 'As well as the biodiversity in this wood, human diversity is as important to us,' Jack told me as I sat looking at the plaque that reads *Gwreiddiau Gobaith*, or Roots of Hope.

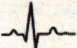

You never forget certain patients or families. Perhaps they are those ones that are most like you at that time. When my daughter was three I cared for a little girl who died in a fire when she was three. The same week Aunty Win died, the first family I broke bad news to lived in the same village, one street away from Win. Often, I have a strong inbuilt desire to find out what happened next in their lives.

A month went by after Luca was taken to London and hundreds more patients passed through the Intensive Care Unit. I would often think about Luca, his wife and his daughter. He was one of those that we as healthcare workers carry along with us. I kept meaning to call London, to find out how Luca was doing, if he had stayed alive. But the endless patients, the pandemic and my life got in the way. Or perhaps I didn't want to know the answer. Many say that it is not the despair that gets them, but the hope that's unbearable. I disagree. For me there is power in uncertainty, because uncertainty contains hope.

I still remember the first time I uttered those three little words. Growing up in a loving Welsh family, I'd heard them countless times. But saying them yourself for the first time is unique. You try to pick the right moment, but sometimes the words come out unexpectedly, catching both you and the listener off guard.

If 'I love you' are the three most important words in life, then 'I don't know' are the most crucial in medicine. Despite their significance, they're seldom used. Their strength lies in acknowledging that doctors don't, and can't, know everything. For me, the first time I confessed my uncertainty to a patient's family was after caring for a young man who died from sepsis. As an ICU doctor surrounded by advanced tests and scans, I still couldn't answer his family's simplest and most important question. Trying to grasp the situation, his mother asked, 'Why him? Why has he died?'

Medical encounters often revolve around unknowns. Patients and families frequently challenge us to predict the future, asking, 'Will she survive?' or 'When can I go home?' Like skilled meteorologists, we blend science, history and intuition to estimate a possibility we hope aligns with the truth.

Consider a weather forecast predicting a 90 per cent chance of rain. If the sky remains clear, the prediction wasn't wrong – truth just resided in that smaller 10 per cent. Being open about uncertainty fosters understanding: a 90 per cent chance of rain may prompt you to take an umbrella, but 'I don't know' initiates deeper, more nuanced conversations.

Looking a patient or relative in the eye and saying 'I

don't know' is challenging. These words are hard to say. It's difficult to admit the limits of our knowledge, and sometimes it means hinting at the boundaries of medical understanding. Patients and families often expect doctors to have definite answers, assuming modern medicine can cure them. It can be surprising when we don't and can't.

These words also carry risks. Standing on the solid ground of reason, it can become slippery when uncertainty melts that foundation. You can falter, become unsteady, and lose your grip. Admitting 'I don't know' can be a disorienting experience for doctors, leading to more profound self-questioning.

Yet these words also hold immense power: the power of hope, suggesting a chance for recovery. They also inspire the pursuit of a better understanding of the unknown. Even when hope fades and answers remain elusive, perhaps honesty with yourself and those you care for is valuable in itself – though I'm not entirely certain. I don't know.

The guessing would soon end. It was at the end of another busy Friday afternoon when a new patient was wheeled into my area of ICU. Arriving by ambulance, they looked thin, weak but were breathing for themselves. Bad timing I thought, right at the end of the day, a new patient, another day when I'll be home late. I caught a glimpse of the back of the patient's head as I walked down the corridor for a handover. I couldn't believe it. It was Luca. Back from London. Back from his death. Even writing these words now makes me smile.

Luca was completely off all life support machines, his eyes open, darting around, trying to make sense of where he was and now who he was. He spoke in Italian then in English. He tried to tell me about the crazy dreams he had been having, first where he was surrounded by lifeless mannequins, another with wasps biting his legs. But the scariest memory was not a dream or delusion at all. It was seeing Big Ben as he was driven back to Cardiff, not knowing why on earth he had been in London or what had happened.

Luca was right to fear the famous clock tower. Officially called the Elizabeth Tower, it lies next to the seat of government, which was the most dangerous place in the UK during the pandemic. Not for those inside, expelling political chicanery and privilege, but dangerous for the safety of the nation after its litany of poor decisions and poor leadership. Luca showed me the last text on his phone from one month ago that still read, 'I won't be in work tomorrow.' Unlike the politicians' messages, this one hadn't been deleted.

As Luca settled into his new temporary hospital home in Cardiff, he rekindled a long-distance relationship with his wife, Aria, like they had years before. This time they weren't separated by an ocean, but by pandemic restrictions keeping the hospital doors closed to relatives. Instead, Luca spoke by video in Italian to Aria, saying he was now much closer to home. As the conversation started to end, I asked if I could borrow Luca's phone. Perhaps for selfish reasons, I wanted to speak with Aria, to help make sense of the story for her and for me. It was a much better conversation than the last time. She cried once again, but this time for all the right reasons. After talking to Aria, I flicked back through Luca's old medical notes on my lap, found the page from a month ago where my tear-smudged word 'hope' still lay. I wondered if I now write not to communicate but to preserve. I turned to a new crisp page and wrote:

> Hi Luca, I spoke to your wife Aria again today. I said how pleased I was that you were back from London after having the life-saving treatment where oxygen was added directly to your blood. You were no longer sick enough to die. There is still a long and winding road to recovery ahead. But for today, you have your life back, your wife has her husband back and your daughter has her daddy back. And I have my hope back.

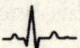

I hardly recognised Luca as he cycled on to the slatted wooden walkway of the cafe suspended over the water where we met. It had been nearly five years since he nearly died. We exchanged small talk about the weather, ordered coffee, argued about who would pay. And then we talked, for hours.

'My life is so different now,' Luca said. "Very different. Better even. I'm glad it happened.'

Luca described how his life before Covid felt like a daydream. He was a passenger on a train of his own life, with scenes from reality flashing by in a blur like my tear-smudged words. Luca's touch with death, getting through the tough recovery that followed and being reunited with his family, meant he now lived for now. He climbed through that train window, jumped into his own life. Luca became acutely aware that he was alive.

'I woke up,' he smiled.

It had been a slow recovery, discharged home in May and returning to work in October. But work too was different.

'There is my actual work as a pharmacist, which I still love. But the most important job I have is working on me.'

This was a novel approach to work for me. I realised that life will always have more to do than time allows. All recorded human history fits into just sixty lifetimes of a hundred years each, making it clear how brief our time really is and how we can never do it all. You are really no big deal. Instead of denting the universe, Burkeman towards the end of his book argues, what really matters is 'making some tiny contribution to the betterment of the environment, or your neighbourhood, or the political culture'.

It struck me that those 4,000 weeks of my life will contain 1,800 weeks in work. Eighteen hundred weeks of work. Boiling your entire career down to these simple numbers may help you to move from last year to the next with a different view of how you relate to time, to people, and to yourself. Not everything that weighs you down is yours to carry. Allow the good days to bring you happiness; the bad ones will bring experience of this short life and even shorter career. The true value of any time-management strategy lies in it helping you to neglect the things that don't really matter.

Luca now realised this. As soon as he got home from hospital, he started consuming books. 'The first book I read when I got home was yours – *Critical*.'

Published just before the pandemic, my first book, *Critical*, pulled back the hospital curtain to reveal the science and stories of my life in the high-stakes world of intensive care medicine. For Luca, reading my words was hard because he had lived through much of the detail. Lived experience, or perhaps died experience. But Luca needed to understand what his body and mind had gone through. Hearing him speak about this over coffee really got to me. I tried not to show it. I had never imagined that the words I wrote in that first book years ago, after meeting other patients like just Luca, would one day mean so much for my future patients. I pulled out a crumpled sheet from my bag that I had photocopied from Luca's notes. It felt right to read out to Luca the words that I had written to him when he was too sick to hear them. After all, I wanted to write to patients and not about them.

'Thank you for writing down my story,' he said after reading them through from top to bottom.

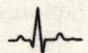

I was looking at a white church in the distance that reminded me how much another storyteller had improved the lives of millions, including my own children, through his stories. One of my favourite questions to ask resident doctors during ward rounds is about the connection between Cardiff, *The BFG* and intensive care medicine. Surprisingly, few know that Llandaff, a cathedral village just a mile from our wards, was home to the world-renowned children's author Roald Dahl. He was born in Cardiff and christened in the Norwegian church in Cardiff Bay where Luca and I were meeting. But Dahl's legacy extends far beyond his literary achievements. His life, marked by personal tragedies, spurred contributions to medical science that often go unrecognised.

Roald Dahl's life, though privileged, was interspersed with profound hardships from an early age. At three, his sister succumbed to sepsis from a ruptured appendix. During the Second World War, Dahl narrowly escaped death when his Gloster Gladiator biplane crashed in the Egyptian desert, leaving him with a broken nose, fractured skull and a concussion. The five years between 1960 and 1965 were particularly harrowing. His three-month-old son, Theo, suffered a brain injury after being struck by a taxi in New York. Then, in 1962, a measles outbreak claimed the life of his 7-year-old daughter, Olivia, after the virus spread to her brain, causing encephalitis. Adding to his woes, his wife, the actress Patricia Neal, suffered a massive stroke while pregnant with their fifth child.

Dahl tackled each crisis with remarkable determination. To manage his son's hydrocephalus, a condition causing fluid accumulation in the brain, Dahl collaborated with hydraulic engineer Stanley Wade and neurosurgeon Kenneth Till. They developed the Wade-Dahl-Till (WDT) valve, a device that significantly improved the treatment of hydrocephalus by preventing blockages in the brain's fluid drainage pathways. This invention continues to benefit patients worldwide.

Olivia's death profoundly affected Dahl, prompting him to advocate passionately for vaccination. *The BFG*, dedicated to Olivia, was published fourteen years after the introduction of the measles vaccine that could have saved her. In 1986, Dahl penned a heartfelt letter urging widespread vaccination, which public health campaigns still use today to emphasise the importance of immunisation.

Dahl's commitment to medical advancements didn't stop there. Frustrated by the inadequate post-stroke care his wife received, he devised an intensive rehabilitation programme that proved instrumental in her recovery. Patricia Neal not only regained her ability to speak and move but also returned to acting, earning an Oscar nomination three years after her stroke. Their innovative approach to stroke rehabilitation laid the groundwork for modern techniques and contributed to the formation of the Stroke Association.

Roald Dahl's story reminds us that a writer can change the world not only through words but through transformative actions. His medical innovations, born out of personal tragedy, continue to save and improve lives, illustrating the profound impact one individual can have across diverse fields.

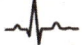

Once Luca had made sense of his own story, he could plan where the plot of his own life would take him.

'After I understood what had happened, I wanted to get better. Better than before.'

After finishing my book, his taste in literature improved greatly. He bought endless self-help books, books on self-development and self-improvement. Books changed not only Luca's internal voice, making him less shy and more willing to speak his mind, but started to transform his body. Waking at 5 a.m. to exercise is now his superhuman ability, hacking the time restraints of being a busy father to not only Sofia, but now his second daughter, Grazia. Words were a fantastic way to do that. Words have power.

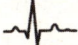

After talking with James Wong at the Hay Festival about the power of greenery, I met another panellist, Professor Neil Frude. As a clinical psychologist obsessed with books, he developed 'bibliotherapy' as a powerful tool in mental health treatment. This innovative approach harnessed the transformative power of literature to provide solace, guidance and a sense of connection to those struggling with psychological challenges.

Frude was not the first to transform the power of books

into a physical reality. Mexican architect-turned-artist Jorge Méndez Blake turned literature into sculpture with his installation art project *The Castle* in 2007. At first glance, the piece appears to be a normal brick wall. A closer look reveals a subtle curved bulge in the middle of the 75-foot-long structure. As your eyes move down from the arched top, the cause of this distortion is a single book placed at the wall's base. Lodged in the mortarless foundation, between the floor and the first layer of bricks, is a copy of Franz Kafka's *The Castle*. With his architectural background and a life-long love of books, Blake pays homage to Kafka by placing his novel at the base, warping the monumental red-brick structure. Words really do have power. This is even more poignant as Kafka only ever wrote privately, never intending his work to be published. It was only after his death that *The Castle* was published by a friend. Blake's art reveals the power of a single book, how small ideas can have a monumental effect even when the words are whispered using a faint, shy voice. The quietest person in the room often has the most to say.

Frude harnessed the physical effects of books in a different way, not using them for art but as practical help for patients. His 'Books on Prescription' project revolutionised how mental health professionals could approach treatment. This government-backed scheme, where doctors could prescribe self-help books instead of pills, was rooted in Frude's extensive research and clinical experience. It still provides cost-effective, accessible and stigma-free treatments. Patients can delve into narratives and advice that resonate with their experiences, offering practical strategies for managing conditions such as depression, anxiety and stress. The books are as effective as the costly pills for mild to moderate conditions, without the side effects.

I've just returned from our annual family trip to Hay Festival. The tradition started when my daughter became obsessed with Julia Donaldson's *The Gruffalo*, but the march of time has morphed her tastes into young adult themes of love, sex and murder.

Just as traditional as the trip itself were the accompanying rain showers, prompting a dash to the undercover deckchairs, where we ate and read, and I started writing this. I was surrounded by words: words of hope for the future, pleas for help from war zones, words seeking understanding, and words that made people smile. These were written and spoken at more than 800 events in eleven days, by 700 people from Bonnie Tyler to Theresa May. Thankfully, there was no dancing. Thousands of books were sold and millions of words were read every day by the 300,000 visitors.

Yet these statistics are dwarfed in just a single day in my own hospital. There are more patient encounters where I work daily than there are events at Hay, more clinics than speeches, more words written about patients than visitors like me on those deckchairs. But medicine often forgets the power of simple words, distracted by the importance of verbal communication skills, simulation training workshops, and human factors courses. These things are important, but let's not forget about the millions of written words that affect patients and staff every day.

I've previously collaborated with the Welsh artist Nathan Wyburn to show the harmful impact that words of hate can have on healthcare staff. In his art installation *Words Bruise* the reddened face of a healthcare worker is formed from hundreds of negative words and phrases sent over social media. But these same staff often use well-intentioned phrases in their everyday work that can hurt patients.

Sadly, familiar terms written in medical notes include 'housebound', 'bed blocker', and patients 'complaining of' things rather than being affected by them. The worst might be 'poor historian', meaning patients who can't give a clear account of their medical history. It is as if we forget that it takes six years of university and a decade of hospital training to become a specialist doctor – and even they struggle to retell a medical history when they're not seriously ill. It's almost as if we're expecting patients to moonlight as a consultant while battling to survive. But my personal nemesis that I'd love to murder (like the plot line of my daughter's latest book) is the 'ceiling of care'. For one thing, care should never be limited, even if treatments are. But what really grates is the idea of a hierarchical escalator of interventions. This suggests that lower-level treatments are somehow inferior to those at the top, and near the ceiling are the 'best' ones.

The truth is that many patients I care for may be treated

with some drugs but not all drugs, many attached to some machines but not all machines. After the complex interplay of wishes and best interests are combined, the conclusion we often reach is that more and more drugs are not better – they would be worse. Similarly, more complex machines wouldn't be the best choice but the worst. And so, not only is the phrase 'ceiling of care' clumsy and poorly formed but it may promote the idea of 'more is better'. Instead, the Australasian approach of describing 'goals of care' is better at describing this complexity, using the same number of words.

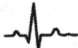

Writing a letter to my Aunty Win was not the first time I'd written a letter to someone very dear. When the Covid pandemic gripped the world, I kept hearing in the media sentiments like, 'Don't worry, it will only kill the elderly, frail or vulnerable.' These people are the core of a society. They are my patients, my friends and my family. Should I not worry about them? Should we just forget about them?

After getting home late from hospital after a long, anxiety-inducing meeting planning our ICU pandemic response, I slid on to an old leather sofa in the jumbled-up spare room of our house, the type of space that acts as a dumping ground for spare chairs and old photo albums. Staring through a window without blinds at the dark sky, I thought about my wife's brother, who is a wheelchair user. I thought about my friends living with cancer. I thought about my parents as they exceed the average life expectancy. I wanted to say something to them, about what the future may hold. I pulled out my laptop, tapped quickly on the keys making countless spelling errors but not stopping. I wrote a letter to them all in just a minute or two, my fingers not lifting once from the keyboard. It was easy to write because it was true and simple and honest. I sent it to my brother-in-law, my parents and my friends by text message before going to bed.

The next morning, I woke to a phone screen filled with missed calls, messages and notifications. My letter addressed to a handful of people had been read by countless more. The world's media arrived on my doorstep and within a week, my open letter to patients during the pandemic was read by over half a million people worldwide and viewed three million times after featuring on television. Bad words grind. Good words mend.

It read:

To those who are elderly, frail, vulnerable, or with serious underlying health conditions,

We have not forgotten about you.

It must be so hard listening to endless news reports that end with, 'Don't worry, this illness mainly affects the elderly, frail, vulnerable, or those with serious underlying health conditions.' What if that is you?

Our passion as an intensive care community is fixing problems that can be fixed. Yet we often meet patients like you who have problems that cannot simply be fixed. As this virus continues to impact on the world, we will meet many more of you. Although we have fancy machines, powerful medicine and talented staff, none of these things cure every disease. All they do is give us time – time to work out what is wrong, time to hopefully treat it, and time for people to get better. But sometimes we already know what is wrong, we already know that there is no effective treatment. And so sometimes the machines offer little, intensive care offers no fix. But hope is not lost. We have not forgotten about you.

As difficult as this is, we will be honest. We will continue to use all of the treatments that may work and may get you back to being you again. We will use oxygen, fluid into your veins, antibiotics, all of the things that may work. But we won't use the things that won't work. We won't use machines that can cause harm. We won't press on your chest should your heart stop beating. Because these things won't work. They won't get you back to being you.

And if these things are still not enough, we will sit with you and with your family. We will be honest, we will hold your hand, we will be there. We will change our focus from cure but most importantly we will continue to care. We have not forgotten about you.

Signed,

The Intensive Care Unit

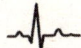

After Luca and I had been speaking for hours, I asked him my last question: 'What would you say to the old Luca, before he was sick enough to die?'

'I would say two things. Firstly, be present in your life. Life can shoot you in the chest. And like being shot, you feel it before you hear it. Life happens without warning or sound.'

Being present doesn't mean you have to own all the problems of the world; often it is a case of 'Not my circus, not my monkey'. But being present allows you to feel your way over uneven ground, as life happens in the cracks.

'And secondly, choose the words you say and read with as much purpose and care as the drugs I dispense at work. Words matter, especially the ones you say to yourself.'

For me, I still write what is hard for me to speak, but important for others to hear. I am lucky that I can do this through my books. But words do not belong only to authors. Anyone can and should write. Start using more written words. Take them inside and allow them to change you. In my science-obsessed, technology-focused world of medicine, it is important to remember that at our core, we are all made of stories. If you cut me in half, next to my organs and my blood, I am filled with words. So are you.

3

RED DUST

Cody, forty years old
Cause of death: Drugs
Cause of life: Live for moments, not things

There are two tough days in any life – the day you realise your dreams cannot be achieved and the day after they have been. Cody's life had everything, yet it meant nothing. So, he disappeared into the red dust of Australia to find something. My life meant everything, yet I too went walkabout to look for something different.

Cody's story has been told many times over since foreign visitors arrived on Australia's shores and decided to call it home. His great-great-grandad had escaped the coal-stained poverty of my home in South Wales for the gold-fractured riches of New South Wales 9,000 miles away. The coal that sustained the Industrial Revolution was called black gold, yet for families digging it from the scarred Welsh ground it brought little shine to their lives. But the yellow gold found in Australia could transform a life of hardship to a life where you get to choose your own future.

Fast forward three generations and an 18-year-old school dropout called Cody also found his riches underground in the mines of Western Australia. History may not repeat but it sure does rhyme. The world's insatiable appetite for new technology led to a lithium rush, found by decimating the homeland of Australia's First Nations peoples. Teenagers like Cody had little reason to study at school when they could instead earn more than their teachers by driving trucks around the ripped-up red dust landscape finding this new white gold.

Cody did make a promise to himself when leaving school – work hard, work smart, keep your head down until you have all the things that his family never had. He imagined the future day when he would be happy – sitting in his nice house, looking at his quarter-acre plot of land, wearing an expensive watch, talking on the latest phone powered by the lithium he was mining, driving a scorched land red truck to his boat, then coming home to a double fridge full of food all while wearing his bright white trainers, downing a cold beer. It would take Cody twenty years of graft to get there. And the day he arrived, soon after turning forty, he died from discovering it still wasn't enough.

I met Cody in the emergency unit of the Royal Perth Hospital. This inner-city hive of ill health is a melting pot of technology, caring staff and social deprivation. The human effects of colonial population exploitation are laid bare for all to see, where drugs, poverty and loss of liberty are as common as high blood pressure. And often the main cause. Despite the turmoil, the hospital's motto 'Servio' is very true – I worked with an incredible group of people who cared about the community, the place and the future. It is an extraordinary place.

Life hadn't always been like this. In school, Cody loved sport. A talented sprinter and basketball player, falling in with the wrong crowd put a stop to that. His life slowly revolved around the five people he was spending the most time with. We often forget the influence that what surrounds us can have on our lives. Think about the people, places or cultures that you are surrounded by, immersed in. They have probably become part of your normal backdrop, the air you breathe. You may have become them. And if you are very different from them, forcing a square peg to fit round holes can end up damaging the peg, not the hole. And think about the conflicts in life, the people you argue with. Sometimes, increasing the distance can quell damage. Or, as George Bernard Shaw said, 'Never wrestle with pigs. You both get dirty and the pig likes it.'

In school surrounded by his crew, soon came the detentions. Then he was dropped from the basketball team. Then a fight turned bad. Then the police. Seeing a poster at the local park advertising a highly paid job, needing only a driving licence, in Australia's mining industry, Cody was in the wrong place at the wrong time.

His job driving trucks around remote mining communities, flying in for three weeks and flying out for one, brought Cody no real satisfaction other than a healthy bank balance. The weeks at home were spent hungover, at all-night parties, spending lots of money and fearing for the next morning. This did bring fleeting pleasures but when the shine had faded from Cody's new gold watch, Cody was lost. He started drinking more and more. Beer turned to spirits. Spirits turned to drugs.

'It was my birthday. I woke up that morning, it should have been the best day. My new truck was delivered, and I was off work for two weeks. I thought I had everything, but then I realised I had nothing.'

So, he drank, smoked, injected, snorted and died in some red dust-covered scrub land surrounded by strangers. Happy birthday. What Cody didn't know is that sometimes when you are in a dark place, you think you've been buried but you have really been planted.

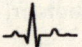

'I have seen many a man turn his gold into smoke, but you are the first who has turned smoke into gold.' These were the words Queen Elizabeth I reportedly said to Sir Walter Raleigh 400 years ago after he introduced tobacco to the English court. This plant, Nicotiana tabacum, which hails from the highland Andes – likely Bolivia or northern Argentina – dates to around 6000 BCE. By 5000 BCE, the Mayans were already incorporating tobacco into their religious rituals – smoking, chewing and even using it as an enema.

Christopher Columbus initially dismissed the value of these tobacco leaves upon his arrival in the New World. It was one of his Spanish crewmen, Rodrigo de Jerez, who recognised their potential in 1492 after discovering them in Cuba. The modern cigarette, as we know it, emerged in 1830 when the South American 'papelate' gained popularity in France.

Our modern relationship with smoking mirrors the ancient practices of the Mayans. For some, it is a quasi-religious ritual, a solace from daily life. Yet tobacco is the most dangerous plant in the world, with smoking standing as the leading cause of preventable death globally. Annually, smoking accounts for nearly 8 million deaths, 10 per cent of which are due to second-hand smoke. Tobacco-related illnesses are responsible for one in five deaths, with smokers typically dying ten years earlier than non-smokers.

Substance misuse accounts for a third of intensive care admissions and 40 per cent of the associated costs. Of these, nearly 15 per cent are tobacco-related, outpacing alcohol at 9 per cent and illicit drugs at 5 per cent.

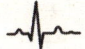

Cody hadn't planned to die. He was just looking for meaning in alcohol, then crystal meth and then cocaine. As the clock of his life ticked on to age forty, like many of us (like me) he had an existential crisis. Many people in their twenties want to be a millionaire. Yet most millionaires want to be twenty again. Working in the intensive care unit, where death is all around me, I'm reminded that the things that matter most are not things at all. For many, it will take an extreme life event or a big birthday to get to this realisation.

The amount of drugs needed for Cody to emulate meaning in his life was more than his heart's coronary arteries could take. His last snort of cocaine melted into the blood vessels in his nose, then sped in Cody's blood stream to his brain's limbic system to produce a fleeting sense of connection. But the drug then arrived at his heart, causing it to clamp down like the rock-crushing machinery Cody drove through the mines. This spasm cut off the blood supply to his overexcited heart that was already hungry for oxygen. Cody had a massive heart attack, a cardiac arrest, and died. As his drinking buddy repeatedly pressed on Cody's chest doing CPR on the 40-degree summer's day, the drug's effects slowly wore off enough to allow his heart to beat again. Twenty minutes later, Cody's struggling body was in the emergency unit where I first met him.

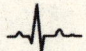

As my life clock ticked past forty, I hadn't planned to emigrate. Our family had many of the modern luxuries at home that Cody had aspired to, albeit without the Australian weather. I loved my job as a doctor and writer. My family were close by, my friends even closer. My wife loved her job teaching in a primary school in the local village. Our daughters were settled in school. We had a dog we loved and a cat that hated us. And all of this meant something. We had meaning. We were safe. Settled. Life was predictably good. And that was the problem.

In his book *Look Again*, the American academic Cass Sunstein argues that a fulfilling life, the so-called good life, is textured by three vital elements: things, meaning and variation.

The tangible 'things' that ground us – our environment, possessions and physical aspects of our daily interactions – are important. These elements offer a comforting consistency, a cornerstone of stability that, much like the life support machine in my intensive care unit, forms the baseline from which we navigate the complexities of existence. This second dimension goes beyond the physical, encompassing our values, beliefs, and the purpose we derive from our connections and experiences. Although there can be no one definition of what meaning means to different people, we all need 'it', whatever it is for us. This meaning doesn't need to be bold or grand. It can be as simple as the small herb garden we tend, the sports team we coach, the job we find fulfilling, the children we care for. However, it's the third element that Sunstein posits as crucial for a vibrant life that made us emigrate – variation. Far from being a risk or a stressor, uncertainty and diversity in experience is an important part of being. This variation isn't just about seeking novelty. It's about enriching our cognitive landscapes and enhancing adaptability. By integrating varied experiences into our lives, we prevent the stagnation of our thoughts and feelings, fostering a dynamic interplay between comfort and challenge.

Like many families, we had emerged from years of lockdowns, uncertainty and restrictions. As well as killing more than 7 million people worldwide, Covid also killed variation for many. During that period, our family had a diary filled with blank spaces where it used to show weekends away and long-haul flights. But some of that time was bizarrely liberating due to the variation it brought, especially with my wife and I working in education and medicine. In many ways, I had never travelled so much or had so much variation. I didn't need my passport for any of these trips: they all took place in my own hospital.

As a new consultant years before, the first thing I did was take a mystery tour of my own hospital. I pressed the top button in the lift, going to the seventh floor, before walking into and out of every corridor I passed. I soon found specialties that I hadn't known existed, equipment I didn't know we had, and people I had never met. I did the same on each floor down until I became subterranean.

Before the pandemic, that hospital tour had faded from my memory. The Intensive Care Unit I worked in had thick walls that were hard to leave, thanks to the protection they gave to patients and staff. And yet, shelter also brings shade. It stops light from shining on new ideas and better ways of working. Covid changed all of that.

We soon found that intensive care was not one location but many. Coming to work was like visiting new places. Again, I travelled around the hospital: to respiratory wards, to the children's hospital, to wherever I was needed; and sometimes to the chapel, where I was not. Again, I spent time with new people as well as old friends, across the rickety bridge between specialties. Cross-disciplinary working meant that we moved between worlds and didn't become so easily frustrated with each other. It wasn't all rosy, of course, but, like making friends on a holiday, we knew that it wouldn't last for ever, so we all made the most of the good times.

These trips around my own hospital, and into the working lives of others, have been hugely valuable. Although I didn't exactly walk in someone else's shoes, at least I now know what shoes they wear and where the shoe cupboard is.

Coming out from the pandemic, we all thought we would go mad with travel plans. Yet the reality was different. Travel was still tough, expensive and overbooked. Life actually became more predictable rather than less. Rather than emulating the post-war boom of the '50s and '60s, our post-Covid life was actually stagnant. The luxury of being too safe. We were bored.

And then an email landed in my inbox during a tough October. That week I'd received a pension tax bill, been shouted at by a stranger for my views on vaccination, done multiple consultant night shifts paid at plain rates, missed my dad's birthday to attend a research conference and prepared for a teaching session that no one turned up for. I wasn't burned out – I still enjoyed my job, my colleagues and the patients. I was instead missing the last piece of a good life: variation. Sometimes radical change is easier than subtle change.

So it was painful to read the opening paragraph of an email promising academic promotion, better conditions, endless sunshine, good coffee and a health system that was doing well. It wasn't really these aspects that were attractive. It was the radical change in itself. This was painful to read because I knew that we had to give it a go. Because it offered variation. The problem was that the job offer was 9,000 miles away, in Australia.

I read this email during a rare time of being forced to do nothing other than think. Although I think I'm a reflective person, the mirror only really comes out when I need to make something out of the reversed image. Perhaps there is something to write or a student to speak with. Reflecting for a purpose can feel sickly. It can be cathartic, but it isn't healing.

So I never expected to have a deeply emotional experience, with a tear in my eye, while sitting on a plastic chair in the middle of a basketball court. But I did. Perhaps it was because I'd just finished a night shift. I'd just spoken with another family where grief had unexpectedly knocked on the door of an otherwise uneventful Tuesday. Perhaps my vagus nerve had reacted to the minor prick from my Covid vaccine booster I had a minute earlier. More likely, it was because I'd just spent an uninterrupted fifteen minutes thinking about how the past year had consumed me, my family, and my whole world.

When was the last time you sat down and did nothing for fifteen minutes? I mean nothing. For me, it was probably when I was ten years old. The second-best thing about having my Covid vaccine was the fifteen enforced minutes when I had to sit down and wait to check there were no side effects, without a phone, with only my thoughts. I did nothing, yet something happened. I was surrounded by Army volunteers and redeployed health staff in the middle of a leisure centre, whose purpose was now more directly linked to health than ever before.

Grasping at nothing is hard, so I started remembering. I remembered the first patient with Covid we had cared for. I remembered the first patient who had died. I saw my fingers pressing the numbers of that first phone call that started and ended with 'I'm sorry'. I also remembered the smiles, the energy of dealing with a new disease, the speed of progress and research, and the tight squeeze of teamwork. I could taste the late-night pizza on the way home from another long shift. Sleeping in another room from my wife and telling my daughters that 'Daddy is safe', not really knowing if it was a lie. I remembered a friend telling me that no day lasts for ever, but then realising that there are a lot of days in a year. But, most of all, I remembered hope.

The hope that not only would tomorrow be better but so too would the day after and the day after that. Even if it wasn't better, it would still be tomorrow.

Finally, I touched my sleeve on the corner of my eye. I hadn't been sure if it was a tear, but it was. Fifteen minutes had passed. I stood up, my plastic chair was wiped down, and the next person sat on it. And then I realised that reflection for reflection's sake can be cathartic and perhaps even healing. And then I replied to the email asking me to go to Australia. 'Yes.'

After long family discussions, complex visa and equivalence processes, tearful leaving parties and packing up our family home, we left. And, after working in Australia, meeting Cody and many others, I can honestly say that most 'things' there were better. The email was right: academic promotion, better conditions, sunshine, good coffee and a health system that was doing well. In fact, there are many things that the NHS could, and should, learn from its distant, sun-kissed cousin. Changes that could help manage the current outbreak of strikes and dissatisfaction in the NHS, whose principles are as important, and as right, as ever. Yet we eventually came home. Why? I'll tell you by the end of this book.

Feeling homesick in Australia, I spoke to good friends by phone that I call my 2 a.m. crew – the people you know will pick up if they see your name on the phone to help no matter why or when. I remember clutching for Wales by watching the actor Michael Sheen perform Dylan

Thomas's *Under Milk Wood* live on stage at London's National Theatre, streamed over the internet. It was a bridge to another place, to my home that felt so far away. And bizarrely one year later, I would be back at home, working as a medical adviser with Michael Sheen as he played the Welsh politician Aneurin Bevan, founder of the NHS, in a play at the National Theatre in London, written by my friend Tim Price. Life is luck. A million lotteries.

It was a role reversal when I met Cody a year after his death. On a bright sunny day in Old South Wales, rare rays of yellow light streaming through the window of my office, speaking on a video call with Cody wrapped in an oversized hoodie during a grey Australian winter. He looked cosy, he looked well and happy. Clean for nine months, his employer had given Cody a second chance. He still had many of the physical things that he had aspired to. But his gold watch was in a box behind him and instead on his wrist was an electric model powered by the lithium he had dug from the ground. Cody needed a watch with a sports mode to help with the rediscovered meaning in his life and the lives of others.

'Getting clean was fine,' he said. 'Staying clean was always going to the tricky bit. That's why I'm now working with kids to stop them getting there in the first place.'

He had learned that life was not a bucket to filled with stuff but a fire to be kindled. The bright white trainers that were sticking off the end of his bed when I had first met Cody had a bigger back story. As a kid Cody loved basketball.

A SECOND ACT

At 6-foot-2, long and flexible, he was a great player, made for the sport. He led his school team, spent the purple-skied evenings at neighbourhood courts, but work soon stole all his time for living. His love for trainers first came from their function on the court. But this morphed into fashion where function was a by-product.

In the time since Cody died, he found an old basketball in his garage and headed to his local court. First, he was alone, missing the hoop far more times than scoring. But soon Cody connected with others who were similarly hanging out. It was here he read the second poster that would change his life. Rather than advertise a well-paying job, this one asked for people's time for free. 'Coach needed for local youth basketball team,' it read. Cody nervously went along the next weekend, lacing up his trainers for their true intention for the first time in years.

'We came third in the whole of WA [Western Australia] last year!' Cody said, with a wide smile, almost allowing himself to be happy, to be proud of something.

But meaning didn't stop there.

'To stay clean, you have gotta pour yourselves into something else.'

So Cody approached the drug rehab centre that had helped him to start their own team. Now every Sunday, a smorgasbord of tall, short, fit, fat, great and terrible players turn up. They rarely win. But they have all won a sense of meaning, no matter how small, to bring life back into their life.

'I can't wait to get back from work away nowadays. I head straight to the court, see how my friends are doing and get coaching. I love it. In fact, I've got a game in ten so I'm going to have to shoot, sorry!' Cody said, looking at his lithium-powered watch. Then he was gone.

4

Summer

Summer, twenty-five years old
Cause of death: Suicide
Cause of life: Be surrounded with good people

Summer still remembers the day she died. Paradoxically, it was also the day that saved her life. She wrote to me after reading *Critical* and we arranged to talk. Sitting on the edge of her bed, wearing a dark jumper over a white shirt with pale porcelain skin and blonde hair wrapped over her shoulder like a scarf, she told me why she had wanted to die. A tattered Hello Kitty doll was perched alongside her after sharing the highs and deep lows of her twenty-five years on Earth. Kitty's delicate stitching was there for Summer to hold on to when anxiety first troubled her at the age of eight, and when her teenage years were stolen by depression and anorexia. Kitty journeyed through mental health units across the country, while Summer's friends swam on sunny holidays and partied in dark nightclubs.

And Kitty was there when Summer took an overdose of prescription pills to end her life. But Kitty was by her side when Summer survived. When she opened her eyes. When she learned how to live a better life, the second life many in her situation don't get to have. And when she told me her story so that you too can benefit from what she learned.

It was in one of her lowest moments that Summer knew what she wanted to do for a career. During one of her stays in a psychiatric hospital, she was cared for by a nurse called Sammy, who was caring, strong, clever – and scarred. Summer recognised the parallel lines on Sammy's left arm. She realised that people like her could still help others despite their own troubles, or even because of them. From that moment, Summer wanted to be a mental health nurse. To turn the helped into the helper.

As she focused on college work, life became more stable. Summer got the grades needed for nursing, found the perfect university course and packed her bags, excited about the future. But that cold October a relationship broke down, university life became harder and Summer's gran died suddenly. She fell back into her old patterns, moved home and entered a downward spiral. On 16 March 2020, as the British prime minister announced a nationwide lockdown, Summer swallowed a fistful of sedative pills. Her mum found her wandering around the house, turning lights on and off, before collapsing on to her bed. The benzodiazepine drugs dampened the brain receptors that keep us aware, conscious, alive. They also relaxed Summer's muscles, preventing her from coughing and eventually from breathing. She was vein-blue when the ambulance arrived. Her heart stopped three times in the emergency department as staff rushed plastic pipes into her lungs and squeezed against her heart by pressing on her ribs. Summer's parents were devastated when doctors told them that their 25-year-old daughter might not survive.

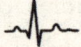

Self-harm is, sadly, one of the most common reasons for admission to an intensive care unit. I have met patients who have tried to die in so many ways. The ripples from these terrible events extend far beyond the individual: we see the impact they have on the families, sitting for hours in lonely waiting rooms, and the nurses caring for them. Suicide is not painless, for staff, for families or for patients.

The chance of dying by suicide depends on where you live, among numerous other factors. According to the World Health Organization, if Antigua is home, you have the lowest chance, at just 0.3 people per 100,000, while southern Africa's Lesotho has the highest rates, at 87.5. Globally, more than 800,000 people kill themselves each year, twice the number who die from murder. Suicide is the leading cause of death in young people (fifteen to twenty-four years old), yet older people are the most likely to die in this way. There are big sex differences too, with the suicide rate for men being double that of women. It is often a fleeting, rash decision. Several peer-reviewed research papers have shown that 70 per cent of survivors thought about killing themselves for less than an hour, with a quarter considering it for just five minutes.*

In one case, the gap between the first impulse to die and the act of jumping from a bridge was only five seconds. Just as many with mental illness are never affected by suicidal thoughts, and not all people who attempt suicide have mental illness. Around half of those who die by suicide have no diagnosable mental health disorder. And for those with mental illness, proper treatment can really help. This is because the majority of people who feel suicidal do not actually want to die. They want the situation they are in to stop, the feelings to go, for life to return. This distinction is small, but critical. Understanding that death may not be the intent in a suicide attempt may mean we can save lives by putting more preventative measures in place.

Let's take the example of death by oven fumes, as was the case for the American poet Sylvia Plath. She ended her life by putting her head into her kitchen oven, carefully placing a towel under the door to protect her sleeping children. This was not unusual in 1963. Death by breathing in oven fumes was used in half of all British suicides until the '70s. Yet this plummeted to zero in just three years.

To understand how, we will meet cows in Chicago and a British Gas pioneer. Soaring electricity prices in the '50s led to factory workers facing redundancy in Chicago's

---

* A summary of these findings can be found https://www.hsph.harvard.edu/means-matter/means-matter/duration/

meat-packing district as cuts ran deep. The union president explained the problem to his refrigerator engineering friend. They hatched an idea to liquefy gas recently found in the Southern Plains and transport it on barges up the Mississippi to reduce costs. It was a success, proving liquid gas as a cheap and safe fuel source.

The talented British engineer Denis Rooke was part of a small team to pioneer sea transportation of this new liquefied natural gas. Son of a south London travelling salesman, Rooke 'came from a simple working-class family'. He spent his childhood in Great Ormond Street Hospital with recurrent illnesses and so was unable to read, write or properly walk until the age of seven. But Rooke developed a love for machines when he returned to school, later graduating from University College London with a degree in mechanical engineering.

After successful pilot journeys in the '60s, natural gas was found in the sea around Britain. With these huge reserves, the decision was made to convert every British consumer appliance to burn this natural gas instead of coal gas that had been used until then. This mammoth task involved the replacement or modification of 35 million units across 8,000 models in 13 million homes.

Under Rooke's leadership, the operation went remarkably smoothly, within budget and the planned ten-year timescale. It was 'perhaps the biggest peacetime operation in the nation's history', with Rooke becoming chairman of British Gas and one of Britain's most distinguished civil engineers.

When he died aged eighty-four, he had been made an Order of Merit by the Queen, joining just twenty-four others including Baroness Thatcher and the Duke of Edinburgh. But what has this to do with suicide?

The conversion of British appliances from coal gas to natural gas, which does not contain carbon monoxide, stopped this form of suicide almost overnight. Amazingly, there was also a dramatic reduction in the overall number of deaths by suicide. Instead of dying by other means, those who had planned to die in their ovens instead continued to live. Fleeting suicidal thoughts were extinguished by the new barrier to death.

And these barriers can be subtle. After three people jumped to their deaths in a ten-day period on the Duke Ellington Bridge in Washington, a physical suicide barrier was erected. Despite a similar bridge being just 200 metres away, the local suicide rate was halved – the exact number that would have jumped from Ellington Bridge. Similarly, in many low- to middle-income countries where self-poisoning with pesticides is more common, bans on pesticides have reduced suicide rates. If we consider that 60 per cent of deaths by firearms in the US are self-inflicted, tighter gun controls there may help protect us from ourselves as well as from others. Out of all the many reasons people are cared for in the ICU, I hope we can get to a world where it is not self-inflicted. The best way to survive the ICU is not to go there in the first place.

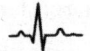

As an early-career doctor, I worked in a friendly, supportive hospital in the small town of Bridgend, South Wales. Sadly, my time there coincided with a spate of teenage suicides in the local community. The boys and girls who were found before death were brought to our Intensive Care Unit. All of them died. A total of twenty young people, with their lives ahead of them, died through hanging in just three months, with twenty families left grieving. In the ICU, we see the sharp side of the global mental-health crisis. In many ways, ICU is simply a hyper-acute department of social services, where the all too real end result of deprivation, poor opportunities, poverty and drugs are written on to patients' bodies.

Sadly, this is not restricted to patients but extends to staff. I've known three colleagues who have tragically lost their battle with despair. Alarmingly, doctors are up to five times more likely than the general population to die by suicide with female and resident doctors especially high risk. Staggeringly, one in twenty-five doctor deaths results from suicide. This risk escalates further for those facing patient complaints.

The colleagues I've lost were outwardly the most cheerful, carefree and seemingly stable individuals. In medical training, we learn to adopt a facade of resilience when dealing with patients' families, but this mask often hides our own need for help. Forgiving ourselves for mistakes is a monumental challenge. It is of course natural and good to look back on your life, but don't stare. These mistakes may not be visible to others, but we carry them deep within us. Despite working in healthcare, we still face the stigma of mental illness, compounded by personal struggles like anyone else. Peering over the brink of life can be a heavy burden for those trying to pull patients back.

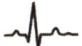

Returning to Summer, as her parents were told their daughter might die, her life flashed before her eyes. She remembers this burst of life as her heart stopped and started and stopped again. She says it gave her a sense of clarity, of what was important. 'People are important,' she tells me, 'not things.' In that flash, Summer didn't see a new iPhone or an expensive dress. She saw her mum, her dad, good friends she hadn't spent enough time with, lying laughing on the grass on a hot day and staying up late to see the stars sink to the horizon.

The 'life flashing before your eyes' scene is so common in films, it is a tolerated cliché, a photo montage of the highs and lows of a life lived. Terry Pratchett put it best: 'It is said that your life flashes before your eyes just before you die. That is true, it's called Life.' In fact, life probably does flash before your eyes in some form as you die. An elderly patient with a do-not-resuscitate order died unexpectedly during a recording of her brainwave activity. A team of neuroscientists analysed the recordings and found an oscillatory brain wave pattern where alpha, beta and theta bands decreased and activity in the gamma band relatively increased. These patterns are typical of memory recall and visions, occurring during meditation, dreaming and even drug-induced hallucinations. So, if life does flash before your eyes, what would be in your flash? Think about it now while you are alive – perhaps it will help make a change.

For some, suicide is not a spur of the moment decision, but a carefully planned event. This extra time can allow for a life review in the form of words rather than visions, a note or letter left behind. Some people write to communicate, some to be honest, and others to preserve a memory of life. Summer wrote a note to say thank you, and sorry:

> 'Mum and Dad, I love you so much, thank you for being there and sorry I couldn't be there for you. Summer x'

It said everything, but was too short, a life reduced to just twenty-two words. Although people with terminal disease have this opportunity too, unexpected death accounts for 10 per cent of those classified as 'natural' and is higher in younger people. So, writing to others when you are well is a great idea. And it doesn't have to be morbid. It can be an opportunity to reappraise what is important to you, what you want to say to others, what you want them to know. It can help you reflect on your life now.

As the dust of death coated healthcare workers during the pandemic, I thought about the possibility of my own death, and what I would want to say to my family if the worst were to happen. Early one morning before my first pandemic ICU shift, I hurriedly wrote a text message to my wife and pressed 'Send' before thinking too much about it. It was easy. The important things were obvious, the irrelevant didn't feature. It read:

Things you should know in case I die:
- I have had a bloody wonderful life. I have found love, travelled, partied, had two fab children, spent time with friends, family and done things I had never dreamed of.
- I love my job even though it can be hard and dangerous. Touching the lives of others is the best feeling in the world.
- Easier said than done, but don't stay sad for too long. Remember the good times, the times we laughed and the times we cried. Look at old photos, remember me on my birthday, but don't stay sad too long. We only have one life, as I now realise. Go and live it – Al, Evie, Mimi, Mum, Dad, Chester. Get out there and make your way with me in your thoughts and memories but not as a weight on your back.
- If I get a 'last wish' it would be:
    A flat white
    Some REM playing
    Some LSD ideally

- I'd like to be buried but don't really mind. A completely non-religious service, but one prayer so my mum and dad feel supported. Ideally, 'Nightswimming' as a song. I would like to be made into a skeleton ideally.

Love you all.

Al, you are the love of my life.

Mum and Dad, you are amazing people and thank you for fighting for me.

Evie, you are a gifted reader and writer. I think you will write a book yourself in the future. Love you to the Moon and back, brush your teeth.

Mimi, you are a marvellous scientist. I think you will help care for people in the future. Remember our funny songs.

See you on the other side if there is one!

Matt x

What would yours say? Would you live your life differently with this in mind?

⎯⋀⎯

Seven weeks after her death, Summer opened her eyes. Intensive care had been rough: plastic tubes in her veins, a tracheostomy, hallucinations in the form of a zombie apocalypse. While ICU brings hope and new beginnings, this life-saving comes at a steep price. Physically, patients who leave the ICU are weakened, with muscles shrunk, energy depleted and even voices altered. Scars – both visible and hidden – mark their bodies. Fatigue can last months, shortness of breath can stay for ever. Their skin becomes dry, their hair can fall out. But the psychological toll can be even more profound. Relationships may strain or break, financial burdens grow and intimate aspects of life, like sexual health, suffer. Anxiety and depression can linger, as patients grapple with a new reality that their time in ICU has shaped. Sleep can be hard to find. The battle for survival is just the start; the journey to reclaim a life once lived is often long and challenging.

Speaking to her mum by video call, Summer burst out crying. Not because she wanted to die, but because, for the first time since she was fourteen, she wanted to live. It was like a switch had been flipped in her brain after seeing the effects her actions had had on others. And when her tracheostomy tube was removed, not only were her thoughts different but so was her voice. Vocal cord pressure had changed her once sweet, melodic tones to a deeper, more confident and solid sound. It was a voice happy to speak her mind and live on her own terms, knowing what mattered in her second life.

Summer told me she was 'no longer a doormat to others, but a speed bump'. Stopping those who didn't want the best for her from running her over and slowing down others, preventing them from coming to harm. She surrounded herself with people who made her 'feel more like herself'. This is important because your personality traits can morph into those of your closest friends. Studies have shown this also extends to behaviour. If your best friend smokes, you are over 60 per cent more likely to be a smoker yourself. If a friend of your friend smokes, you are still nearly 30 per cent more likely to smoke. And for a friend of a friend of a friend, the likelihood is 10 per cent. And so goes the Mexican saying, 'Show me who you're with, and I'll tell you who you are.' Sometimes people in your life may not be good for you. We instinctively tend towards solutions that involve adding something rather than subtracting, even when subtraction would be better.

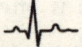

So what does Summer's second act look like? Well, not everything is great all of the time. Good days bring her happiness, and bad ones now bring experience rather than doom. 'Not everything that weighs you down is yours to carry,' she says. Having seen the worst that life can offer, Summer feels this time is a bonus. 'We all will have terrible days, loss, sorrow and heartbreak. But there will also be happiness, contentedness, joy. In the end, everything happens to everyone. Expect it, it is what it is.'

Summer explains what would have helped her in those dark times. And it wasn't practical advice or solutions. 'If you know someone in your life is in trouble, you don't always need to give them answers. Just being there can be enough. It is everything.' Listening, holding and breathing with someone in trouble can make an enormous difference. Sit in the rubble with them. Don't feel you have to solve their problems, just listen. People don't always want advice. They often know what they should be doing. They want someone to be there while they try.

I ask about the future, what goals Summer has. She half-smiles. 'Life is not a game of top scores, or a league table. I'm trying to live for the next few moments, not too many more.' The toughest times in my own life were when I couldn't achieve what I had always hoped or just after I had. The opposite of happiness is not failure, but boredom. I now try to do whatever comes next rather than chase what should be next. Because time is tight and fleeting.

I asked Summer how I could protect the people I love, especially my two daughters as they grow up, navigate friendships, social media, body image. 'Take them to one side tonight and tell them if they ever need you, no matter what they have done or how bad a situation they are in, you will be there. No matter what. No questions. Anytime. Day. Night. You will be there to listen, to hold them, to help them, to help them pick-up the pieces.' I did just that.

In the years that followed Summer's cardiac arrest, she fought against intrusive thoughts circling her mind from her time in intensive care. They would often creep up on her or sometimes jump out from behind the door – vivid, haunting memories of her journey back to life. Some days it was the relentless beeping of monitors, others the sterile scents or feelings of helplessness, leaving her trapped in an endless loop of anxiety and fear. But she got through them – by playing the computer game Tetris.

Tetris is a classic puzzle video game where players manipulate falling geometric shapes to create complete horizontal lines on a grid. The player rotates and positions these shapes as they fall to fill gaps, forming solid lines. When a line is completed, it disappears, making room for new shapes. The game increases in speed and difficulty as it progresses, challenging us to think quickly and strategically, avoiding the building stack of shapes from reaching the top of the screen. This takes a lot of brain work, using parts of the brain that co-ordinate and file memories in the right places.

Tetris was designed in 1985 by Russian computer scientist Alexey Pajitnov while working for the Soviet Academy of Sciences. Pajitnov named the game by combining 'tetra' (meaning 'four') and his favourite sport, 'tennis'. Despite selling more than 500 million copies, Pajitnov has no income from the world's most popular game as the copyright was retained by the Soviet state. But that is not why he made the game. Pajitnov, from behind the Iron Curtain, thought games could bridge the gap between logic and emotion. And twenty-five years later he would be proved right after his game helped Summer and countless colleagues of mine working in intensive care.

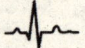

In the wake of the pandemic, my friend Dr Julie Highfield had her work cut out. As a consultant clinical psychologist, waves of ICU staff queued to see her as they struggled to sleep, were troubled by memories of patients they had cared for and kept replaying scenes of devastation from the tough times.

'Staff did their best to rally and do the job, and quickly became overwhelmed. They were frazzled, at the extreme end of stress,' she told me. But Julie's small team of psychologists in the ICU I worked at couldn't help everyone. She did help me. I spoke with Julie after moving to Australia, feeling particularly homesick during a long run of shifts in a rural hospital. I didn't want to show her that I was missing Wales and so when she asked how I was, I put on a happy face said everything was great and that I was watching a recording of Michael Sheen in Dylan Thomas's *Under Milk Wood* as the sun set. It is never a good idea to hide your feelings from a psychologist, or a friend, and especially not both.

'Oh wow – you really are homesick, aren't you?' she said without a blink. She was right of course. As she was also right to be worried when the pandemic hit not only about patients, but about staff.

'People didn't have their usual ways of coping, their usual outlets. They needed to take time off and those who ploughed on were left with a lot of difficult memories, complicated stories that they are carrying in their minds, weighing them down, burdening them,' she said, reflecting years later.

That's when she agreed to help with a surprising study led by Professor Emily Holmes from Uppsala University in Sweden. Holmes had spent decades studying how using games like Tetris, which use brain regions important for laying down memories, may help people suffering from post-traumatic stress disorder (PTSD). Perhaps this could help the staff relying on Julie.

There are several trauma-focused therapies recommended for PTSD. One evidence-based technique is Eye Movement Desensitisation and Reprocessing (EMDR). In traditional EMDR therapy, patients focus on traumatic memories while moving their eyes in specific ways, such as following a therapist's finger. This process helps rewire the brain's response to bad memories, reducing their emotional intensity. Professor Holmes has used similar underlying theory from EMDR in her novel research of playing visuo-spatial games to interrupt intrusive memories that form after psychological trauma. She had previously used an adapted Tetris game in patients experiencing trauma but it had never been used in the real world.

'People would have intrusive memories – pop-up images, fragments of memories that pop into the mind – making it hard to work and impacting their thinking,' Julie said.

The game requires significant visual and spatial attention, engaging the brain in a way that prevents it from deeply processing traumatic imagery. This competition for cognitive resources can diminish the vividness and emotional impact of traumatic memories. The repetitive and structured nature of Tetris, with its falling blocks and need for quick, strategic placement, serves as a form of bilateral stimulation similar to EMDR. By playing Tetris, and particularly focusing on rotation of the blocks in their mind, patients may provide their brains with tasks that could compete with the mental space used by traumatic recollections allowing cognitive reprocessing.

After four weeks of playing Tetris in this directed way, staff working during Covid went from having fourteen intrusive memories per week to just one per week. It had worked. It wasn't just as simple as playing the game. The participants needed careful assessment and monitoring to target specific memories. Staff were told to use their minds eye to rotate blocks around as they fell. But the principle remained – something as fun and silly as Tetris can help us deal with dark times. Other studies have since shown that Tetris can even physically change the size of brain regions that deal with emotions, such as the hippocampal volume in male soldiers with combat-related PTSD.

And it certainly transformed Summer's mind. After having just three sessions of EMDR and playing Tetris she flew through her first year in nursing training.

'Getting through these memories has had a hugely positive impact on my daily life. I'm now coming to the end of the final year of my nursing studies, the end is in sight. And I can't wait to help others do what I have done.'

It is not just Russian-designed computer games that can help us reconsider and reprocess our life. Board, card and puzzle games played in groups all offer mental health benefits along with social bonding, as supported by numerous studies. These games stimulate cognitive functions, enhance problem-solving skills and provide a structured environment for social interaction, contributing to overall mental well-being.

Engaging in games can reduce stress and anxiety. Older adults who regularly played board games exhibited improved cognitive functions and lower levels of depression. These activities require strategic thinking, memory and concentration, which can keep the mind sharp and mitigate cognitive decline.

Socially, group games foster connections and enhance relationships. Playing co-operative games can increase trust among participants. The shared experience of playing together helps build camaraderie, improve communication skills and create a sense of belonging. This is particularly important in combating feelings of loneliness and isolation.

Furthermore, family game nights or group gaming sessions provide a platform for intergenerational bonding. Families who regularly engage in board games report stronger relationships and better family cohesion. These games offer opportunities for meaningful conversations and laughter, strengthening family ties and creating lasting memories.

So even in 1985 when designing Tetris, Alexey Pajitnov was right. He said then that 'games allow people to get to know each other better and act as revealers of things you might not normally notice, such as their way of thinking'. They have even helped to save the lives of people like Summer. I think we should all play more games.

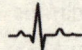

Summer

One year after dying, Summer spotted a crowd of people near her house while driving home from university. Her neighbour lay still on the grass, not breathing, his heart not beating. He, just as she had been, was in cardiac arrest. Like her, he had taken an overdose. One year after Summer's heart was restarted by a stranger, she now tried to save a life. Pushing on his chest as she had been taught in nursing school, Summer tried to give someone else a second life.

When he couldn't be saved, Summer sat with his wife, an arm around her shoulder, not with answers, just with her presence. Summer had come so far, and this seemed the end of a circle, the start of something new. A week after we spoke, Summer started her last year training as a mental health nurse. Right now, she will be putting arms around so many others, helping with her words, her hands as well as with her history.

She revisited the bed in ICU where she woke up. She could see that younger version of herself lying there, sad, in need of healing. 'But I felt like I was grieving for someone who I could no longer find. Now I feel more alive than ever. My second act is the performance of my life.

'There is only a moment between the past and the future. That moment we call life. Don't miss it,' she told me, holding Kitty against her chest.

5

DROWNING NOT WAVING

Mike, fifty-eight years old
Cause of death: Drowning
Cause of life: Together, we are stronger

Mike didn't go fishing to catch fish. It was a slice of time carved out from his everyday life and his everyday job in the insurance industry. Despite there being no Wi-Fi on the ebbing tide between the land and the sea, being here gave Mike a sense of connection. He didn't go fishing to catch fish, but he also didn't go to drown.

Mike first held a fishing rod aged eight during a family holiday to the Isles of Scilly. There he caught his first fish — a brightly coloured wrasse, dark cyan, green and blue with purple accents. Fifty years later, Mike himself turned purple as he was swept away by a wave hitting Wales's rugged coast.

On a grey October Saturday, Mike's wife and children had plans. It was a perfect excuse for him to make a solo fishing trip. He drove two hours towards the coast, picking up a sandwich for his lunch, one that he would never eat. The tidal estuary at Ogmore (meaning 'swift surge') was Mike's favourite spot for bass fishing. He purposely chose a deserted spot away from the concrete causeway, wet and as grey as the sky. He felt nicely alone. Not lonely, but solitary. He would soon learn that we are seldom really alone, rarely an island even when at sea, that we all need a community of strangers around us to live even if we are not drowning. Because Mike hadn't noticed the woman walking her dog near the shore, or the friends who played water polo together parked on the headland above, or the tall, strong man who happened to be a CPR instructor, walking on the beach. He didn't notice the wave that swept him off his feet and caused him to drown.

I met Alicia, one of the people who would save Mike's life. Storm Isha was battering the UK as we spoke, helping to bring her story to life.

Alicia really was a water baby, starting swimming lessons at just six weeks old. As she grew up, her parents drove her to the local swimming pool five times a week to train as a competitive swimmer. At fifteen Alicia's coach, who had played water polo at the Olympics, introduced her to the sport. She quickly fell in love with water polo, joining the Welsh squad soon after university.

Alicia joined the police as a civilian forensic officer. She specialised in CCTV analysis, helped by her photography skills, which she'd gained by taking photos of her friends playing in bands. For all of these reasons, Alicia was the perfect person in the perfect place the day Mike went fishing.

Similarly to Mike, Alicia had grabbed a sandwich for lunch before driving with her friend Amy, a fellow water polo player and physiotherapist, to look at the sea. But Alicia's special skills in noticing tiny changes in scenes, honed by her police CCTV work, played a very different role that day. Sitting in the car park with Amy, overlooking the sea and about to bite into her sandwich, Alicia noticed a tiny dot in the ocean far away.

'Wow, look how high the estuary is . . . what's that man doing? Is he waving?'

> Nobody heard him, the dead man,
> But still he lay moaning:
> I was much further out than you thought
> And not waving but drowning.

These lines are taken from Stevie Smith's poem 'Not Waving but Drowning'. Its central metaphor, mistaking a drowning man's desperate signals for waving, encapsulates a truth about human suffering and misinterpretation. Perhaps a lived experience of the author after her mother's death when she was just sixteen years old.

Unlike the dramatised flailing in movies, drowning is typically silent and subtle. Calling for help is difficult as you struggle to breathe. But so too in many forms of mental health issues or personal crises. Much like the silent drowners, cries for help are often misunderstood or overlooked by those around. Yet in other circumstances, people can bring attention to their plight or issues, not to shine a spotlight on them but as a call for help.

Both perspectives converge on a critical insight: the importance of looking beyond appearances to understand the true nature of someone's experience. Just as recognising the real signs of drowning requires knowledge and attention, so too does recognising the nuanced signals of someone in emotional or psychological distress. Smith's poem serves as a reminder that what appears as attention-seeking may, in fact, be a desperate plea for help, urging us to listen more closely and look more deeply into the lives of those around us.

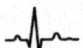

Mike would not be the first person that Alicia had saved from the water. When Alicia was just eleven years old, her younger sister became trapped under an inflatable structure at a local swimming pool. Flipping it over, Alicia saw her sister's gasping face just in time.

A second glance at Mike's distant face a few seconds after she first noticed his waving confirmed her worries. He looked like her sister had years ago. And then he was gone. Mike had been swept out to sea by unusually high rainfall, a strong tide and a huge wave. He was drowning.

A SECOND ACT

Alicia threw her sandwich into the back seat and burst out from her car. There was a woman running up the slipway, wearing a bright yellow coat and waving her arms towards her. This was the last thing Mike remembers seeing. The woman in the yellow coat had already called the coastguard but no one knew how long they would take.

Alicia was used to seeing trauma in her day job with the police, sometimes having to watch recordings of people dying on monitors and video screens. But today it wasn't a recording. She could do something about it. Arriving at the end of the slipway, and now breathless herself, Alicia could see Mike's purple, lifeless body drifting further from shore. The sea was as familiar to her as the swimming pool. She had done a long sea swim in the same area only a few weeks before. And seeing the coastguard's boat still at the launch site around the headland, Alicia knew that waiting for them would be too late to save Mike. He had stopped moving and his purple skin had turned to grey black. Alicia became one of many strangers who would save Mike's life that stormy day.

She pulled off her coat and boots then waded into the biting cold ocean in jeans and a T-shirt. As Alicia battled the waves, another stranger reached Mike at the same time. They pulled his stone-heavy body towards the shore, but with water filling his waders they made little progress. Then from the shore stepped forward a tall, muscular man, who managed to drag Mike's body on to the sand. As Alicia coughed on the seawater she had taken in, her friend Amy sprang into action. She led the CPR efforts, telling people to rotate and press harder or quicker or slower. Many around her thought it was too late. Mike's lifeless body looked dead. And it was. But we'll see the power of hope in many of the stories in this book. And sometimes sheer bloody-mindedness is what can sustain someone and bring them back for a second act.

Nirmal Purja, the Nepali mountaineer and former British Special Forces Gurkha soldier, gained international recognition for his extraordinary achievements in high-altitude mountaineering. He did things that many felt were impossible, all because he refused to give up. He is most famous for his 'Project Possible' campaign, in which he aimed to climb all fourteen of the world's 8,000-metre peaks in a single season. Most said it just couldn't be done. That is when his bloody-mindedness was put into words. In the documentary *14 Peaks: Nothing Is Impossible*, he is shown giving a motivational speech to other mountaineers, in which he says: 'Sometimes you feel like you are fucked, but when you say you are actually fucked, you are only like about 45 per cent fucked.'

In 2019, Purja successfully completed Project Possible, summiting all fourteen peaks in just six months and six days, shattering the previous record of nearly eight years. He found hope when there was little and so, to him, Mike was only about 45 per cent fucked. Alicia was similarly bloody-minded. When many thought Mike had died, she focused on hope.

After the stranger, who Alicia called 'the Mountain Man', finished dragging Mike to shore, he took over doing high-quality chest compressions at Amy's instruction. He was very good at it, not least because he was actually a CPR instructor. Nothing happened for what seemed like ages, until suddenly a gush of cloudy seawater poured from Mike's mouth. But yet another person from the village of strangers was needed to save Mike.

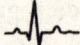

But you don't need to be a CPR instructor to save a life. You just need to finish reading this chapter. The history of cardiopulmonary resuscitation (CPR) is a colourful journey through time, filled with quirky methods and remarkable innovations that have shaped the life-saving techniques we rely on today.

In the 1500s, resuscitation methods were more imaginative than effective. Techniques included using fireplace bellows for 'fumigation with tobacco smoke'. Now that would be a bad idea even when the smoke is directed towards the lungs, but the recommended technique was to administer it rectally to revive drowning victims. Needless to say, few lives were saved despite the Royal Humane Society, founded in 1768 to help drowning victims, installing smoke enema kits along the River Thames. It did birth the phrase 'blowing smoke up your ass', and they even published a rhyme in 1774 to help doctors remember what to do:

Tobacco glyster, breath and bleed.
Keep warm and rub till you succeed.
And spare no pains for what you do;
May one day be repaid to you.

By the nineteenth century, humane societies across Europe were establishing better protocols to revive drowning victims. These methods often involved warming the body and stimulating breathing. External cardiac massage was first reported in 1892, although it didn't become accepted practice until the '60s. Pressing in the middle of the breastbone literally pushes and then pulls blood in and out of the heart. While the compression of the heart between the breastbone and the spine squeezes blood out, the changes in pressure around the lungs then sucks blood out from the heart. High-quality CPR can eject around a third of the normal output of blood from the heart.

Then in 1958 Brooklyn-born William 'Wild Bill' Kouwenhoven combined CPR with his passion for electricity. His fascination was originally sparked by railway linemen dying from abnormal heart rhythms after receiving electric shocks. Despite Glen Campbell's romantic version of working on the telephone exchange wires in the high plains of the Oklahoma in his song 'Wichita Lineman', it was actually a very dangerous job. Kouwenhoven worked out that these deaths were due to an abnormal pattern of cardiac electrical discharge. Rather than the linemen's heart chambers contracting in a neat sequence allowing blood to be ejected, the cardiac muscle would frantically dance around in a useless fashion. Today we call this ventricular fibrillation, or VF. Applying an electrical DC current sufficient to reset this faulty circuit, yet not too high that it would damage the heart tissue, can revert a heart's rhythm back to normal.

Today, using electricity can form a key part of resuscitation along with external cardiac massage when abnormal heart rhythms are present. The widespread adoption of automated electric defibrillators (AEDs) allows the public to not only provide essential bystander CPR but also apply electricity safely to these abnormal rhythms. These self-contained machines automatically assess for deranged electrical signals, resetting them safely with a controlled electric shock. The Danish word given to this equipment, *hjartstarter*, gives a great description. AEDs can even be delivered by drones to remote areas, allowing lives to be saved where the delay waiting for an ambulance to arrive would prove fatal.

But as well as the 'C' part, there is also the 'P' in CPR, which stands for 'pulmonary', or artificial breathing and oxygen delivery to the lungs. The ancient Babylonian Talmud includes a story in which a lamb with an injury to their neck was rescued by making a hole in their windpipe by inserting a hollow reed. Mouth-to-mouth breathing was first described in the Old Testament, where the prophet Elisha saved the life of a young boy by placing his mouth on to the mouth of the child. Sadly, this sensible approach made way for new techniques including rolling patients upside-down in a barrel after water submersion. Unsurprisingly, this was not terribly successful and (hopefully) is no longer used.

It was surgeon William Tossach who first published in a medical journal about mouth-to-mouth when, on 3 December 1732, at Alloa in Scotland, he resuscitated a coal-pit miner. The worker had been 'in all appearances dead' after being carried up 34 fathoms (60 metres) from the bottom of the Scottish coal mine before Tossach 'applied my mouth close to his, and blowed my breath as strong as I could'.

After the discovery of atmospheric oxygen, mouth-to-mouth was stopped due to concerns that exhaled breath was 'empty'. This is true to some extent, although our exhaled oxygen content of 16 per cent compared with atmospheric 21 per cent remains enough to save a life. Instead, arm-lift methods of artificial ventilation were used and even included in Arthur Conan Doyle's short story 'The Adventure of the Stockbroker's Clerk'. After Sherlock Holmes discovers a business owner hung from the neck by his braces, Dr Watson successfully performs the chest-pressure arm-lift, saving the man's life. The practice continued to be recommended until the '60s.

After studies involving thousands of cardiac arrest patients, we now know that chest compressions alone done by the public are more beneficial for most adult victims than combined with rescue breathing. This is because compression-only techniques reduce pauses to blood flow. While there are exceptions, it is only when specialists arrive that more advanced techniques for artificial breathing will now be used.

Drowning can cause a cardiac arrest in several ways. First, our bodies have an instinctive gasp reflex when submerged, especially in cold water. This sudden big inhalation can suck in a full breath of water into our lungs, leading to hypoxia, where the body is deprived of oxygen. Then our body's ancient response to cold water, known as the 'mammalian dive reflex', can slow the heart rate drastically, especially when our face is submerged. In some other cases, laryngospasm —where the vocal cords suddenly close — can prevent water entering the lungs but also blocks air, causing asphyxiation. Finally, even after rescue, secondary drowning can occur when water in the lungs causes delayed respiratory complications like swelling or infection.

The coastguard's lifeboat screamed on to the shore, carrying a nurse from the hospital where Mike would later be taken, who volunteers for rescue service. She added to Mountain Man's CPR with oxygen and rescue breaths using medical equipment. Next an ambulance arrived, and Mike coughed up more seawater, moving and twitching as he tried to breathe. Mike remained critically ill but was on his way to hospital as Alicia peeled off her muddied jeans. Amy patted her bleeding feet, which were cut up from the sharp rocks. Turning on the heating in her car, Alicia stretched back to reach her sandwich from the back seat, wiping down the BBQ sauce from the seat. 'Shall we go home then?' she said to Amy.

Mike had been given a chance at a second act thanks to a collection of people. The woman in the yellow coat who had called the coastguard, Mountain Man who had done CPR, the volunteer nurse in the boat, the stranger who had also gone into the water, Amy the physiotherapist, and Alicia. Even more people would then care for Mike in the intensive care unit. He had gone fishing for solitude but was saved thanks to a crowd. It is easy to forget in today's society of digital solitude that we all need a village of strangers, every day, even when we are not drowning or dying. You can't make a toaster without them . . .

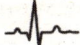

Thomas Thwaites was not a typical student. Yet the questions he asked affect each of us in life and in death. During his time studying design in London in 2010, Thomas didn't restrict his projects to conventional challenges. Instead, he used design to answer more fundamental questions asked by generations before: What does it mean to be human? Can we exist alone?

Thomas decided for his final master's design project to build a toaster. His choice of a toaster as an aim was genius – an object emblematic of modern convenience and individualism. But Thomas didn't want to make a toaster by ordering parts and putting them together. No buying tiny electrical components or even copper wires. He wanted to make a toaster from scratch. And I mean from scratch. Thomas wanted to mine any raw materials and engineer all the parts from first principles.

First, Thomas turned rocks and sludge into materials. Although a modern toaster, costing just £3.94,* has 400 different parts and is made from 100 constituents, Thomas turned his rocks and sludge into just five: steel, nickel, plastic, copper and mica. Steel was made from iron dug from a mine in Wales. His smelting method employed a microwave and a leaf-blower. He extracted copper from run-off water from a deep underwater cave, fashioning the resulting red metal into pins of an electric plug. Mica from cliffs in Scotland acted as a primitive insulator and plastic made from potato starch was moulded using a hollowed-out tree trunk.

Nine months later, standing on the table in his kitchen was something that looked like a cross between a medieval torture device and a loaf of bread. It had cost over £1,500 and seconds after being plugged in, exploded and melted. No toast was made. In an even more barmy project that followed called 'How I Took a Holiday from Being Human', Thomas lived among goats in the Alps, using prosthetic legs and eating grass using an artificial stomach. The toaster may have been a failure, but it was put on display in the Victoria and Albert Museum in London, for Thomas had succeeded in answering a fundamental question.

* This was for the Argos Value Range 2-Slice White Toaster at the time of the project in 2010.

The toaster project was an important journey, illustrating our profound reliance on community and the collective wisdom forged through generations. But this doesn't, and shouldn't, mean that life is all milk and honey. Living shouldn't be easy and convenient with no rough edges. In fact, as Oliver Burkeman describes in his BBC Radio 4 series *Inconvenient Truth*, a comfortable life can be an unfulfilled life.

The limitless progress and reduction in the friction of existence carries risks as well as benefits. Ordering a pizza now needs just a swipe on an app. This feels like progress. But the loss of that slightly awkward conversation with a stranger by phone with a misheard postcode is a minor primer to the bigger annoyances that life will throw at you in the future. Burkeman suggests we should sometimes choose the less convenient option, choose the human interaction. Because these are not really that awkward in the first place and bring with them connection and engagement! Inconvenience is even sometimes part of the reward through these smaller interactions. Discomfort can grow like a muscle; strength you will one day need for the really discomfiting experiences that define life. People are inconvenient.

And, in fact, seemingly convenient approaches are often more inconvenient. The 'unexpected item in the bagging area' at supermarket self-checkouts or the mobile phone app that has replaced your bank but doesn't recognise your face are common examples. Extreme convenience, seen through the long lenses of life, can make life worse.

Maybe this is why I love working in ICU. The struggle and the sadness are the hard bits that also make the highs, the times when people pull through, even better. So next time you are in a restaurant, order by talking to staff not pressing the app, walk past the self-service counter to have inconvenient small talk at the supermarket till and ring for your pizza delivery, knowing that your order may not be quite right – but it will taste better regardless.

No man is an island can be translated into 'no man can build a toaster'. And even if he could, it is less fun than doing it together. Drinking with a stranger is better than drinking alone. It is a parable of modern civilisation's intricacies, our under-appreciated interdependencies, and the lengths one might go to to understand where we fit within the grand tapestry of human achievement. It is about the invisible village of strangers that carry us every day, unseen, unheard and unthanked. Mike was saved on the beach that day by such a group of strangers, all coming together for a very human purpose. Although he went there to be alone, he left alive because he was surrounded by others.

Thomas himself was created by a community of strangers. Although born in England to a children's author mum and professional DIYing dad, he had distant family who had emigrated to New Zealand in the nineteenth century. Upon arrival, these pioneers found themselves in a land both beautiful and daunting. Their survival hinged not on individual prowess but on the collective effort of communities formed by people who were once strangers. These early settlers, bound by shared challenges, built a network of mutual aid and generosity. Neighbours, regardless of origin, became akin to family, sharing what little they had – be it food, tools or knowledge of the land. This spirit of communal support and kindness became the bedrock upon which they carved out their new existence, transforming wilderness into home. Through collaboration with a community of strangers, Thomas's family survived and thrived, laying the foundations for his future exploration into this need for others through the story of a toaster.

From metallurgists to electrical engineers, our lives are enriched and sustained by the invisible threads connecting us to farmers, doctors, artists and countless others. So too, the 'toaster project' is a poignant reminder of our shared humanity, underscoring that the strength of our society lies not in rugged individualism but in our collective vulnerability and collaboration. In fact, our greatest achievements are not solo endeavours but the fruits of communal effort and shared vision, compelling us to acknowledge and cherish our place within the vast mosaic of community.

And even when the community cannot or will not answer difficult questions, this still has value. Often, people don't actually want advice or a problem to be solved. They already know what they should be doing, know the solutions. Often people want instead people to listen and support them. Our strength and survival as a species are not predicated on the individualism celebrated in many modern myths but on our ability to collaborate, share knowledge and stand on the shoulders of those who came before us. So let us stop. Don't try to reach the top by standing on other people. Or put in another way, Thomas's toaster project was inspired by a quote from Douglas Adams's 1992 novel, *Mostly Harmless*:

'Left to his own devices he couldn't build a toaster. He could just about make a sandwich, and that was it.'

And do you know what, that is a very good thing.

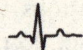

One month after Mike drowned, the village of strangers who gave him another life were reunited. A small gathering at the coastguard's building had been arranged with Mike's family. Although Alicia knew Mike had lived, she was unsure what life was now like for him. She had been told by the coastguards about people they had previously rescued who were left with severe ongoing care needs. Had he been in the water too long to make a complete recovery?

Although she had a tough exterior, her worries about that day manifested in poor sleep and a severe migraine. But Alicia struggled through and just about made it to the event. Entering the room, she first saw Mountain Man, then the woman in the yellow coat and a group of people who she guessed were Mike's family. But there was no Mike. Before she had time to ask, Alicia heard a voice behind her. 'Started without me, have you?!'

Mike's journey to his second act had been tough. A week in the intensive care unit, with very sore ribs thanks to the efforts of Mountain Man, and then a long recovery at home, with recurrent dreams about and flashbacks to the event. Too often we retain the memories we would rather forget, and lose the ones we most want to remember. Mike was back at work, but it had probably been too soon. After an emotional embrace, Mike said thank you to Alicia for saving his life and told her that he had returned to fishing just two months after his cardiac arrest. His wife now wishes him well by saying, 'Drive carefully, don't drown.' The first time he fished again, a shallow stream of water flowed across his boots, and he had a tingle up his spine. But he was soon back to his solo ventures knowing he is always surrounded by a village of strangers. Alicia too returned to her open water swimming, being back in the ocean around the lifeguard station the following spring. The BBQ sauce stains are still on her back seat. As they left the reunion, Mike said, 'I'll never give up fishing, but I have given up drowning.'

6

A Heart in a Jar

Jen, thirty-four years old
Cause of death: Heart failure
Cause of life: Vitam vive, live life

I met Jen's heart six weeks before I met the rest of her body. It was suspended inside a glass container in a museum in London. Jen is the only patient in this book whose heart never did restart after it stopped. Instead, she needed to be gifted someone else's heart to live life.

I met the rest of Jen on a sunny winter's day. She looked the picture of health – a white smile, warm cheeks, soft curls sitting on shoulders covered by a cosy blue jumper. The sun streamed through the large panel windows of her house overlooking the sea on England's rugged south coast.

'Where to start, where to begin,' Jen said. 'It's been an interesting life.'

'Interesting' is one word, but closer to reality would be 'tough'. Jen can't remember a time before her mum was sick. And with her botanist dad exploring the world for the Natural History Museum, her childhood was spent on a tightrope. And then her mum died. Jen was just thirteen. Her world and everything around her turned to rubble. And that was before Jen found out that she had the same heart condition as her mum. And before Jen was told she needed a transplant, the operation that had killed her mum.

Jen's mum first knew something was wrong after fainting on the school bus. Years passed filled with frequent visits to the hospital but by her mid-twenties little more could be done to treat her heart failure. After marrying while still studying at Cambridge University, Jen's parents struggled to have a family despite her mum being told that having children could kill her. Jen was born three months premature at the edge of survival. By the time Jen was ten, her mum couldn't leave the house. Family walks to the pub for a Sunday roast morphed into Jen having frequent sleepovers with friends as her mum spent more time in hospital than at home.

Days after turning thirteen, there was an important phone call. Jen knew it was significant because her absent dad was at home after cancelling a long-planned trip to the Mayan ruins. Hushed voices spoke, bags were packed, tablets were gathered into a bag. Jen was told to hug her mum and then they left for the hospital.

'It felt different. I knew something bad was happening, but no one told me what.'

Three days later, when Jen and her brother got home

from school, her dad and grandmother were waiting at home, clutching cold cups of tea.

'Mum is dead.'

Jen's mum Sally had died on the operating table during a heart transplant. It was a last-ditch attempt to cure very advanced heart failure that we now know was caused by a rare inherited disease; a genetic condition affecting only the female side of the family.

Sally had been a fearless woman. She loved life, wouldn't be told what to do and always put her family first. She had waited until she needed oxygen and a wheelchair before agreeing to a transplant. She knew how high the risks were and knew what it may mean for her two children.

Despite Sally's love, life also stopped for her children after her sudden death. No more ballet. No more horse riding. No visiting other family members or even talking about mum. Jen went back to school the Monday after Friday's funeral. And school was tough. Although taught by nuns who were very familiar with the pain of loss, no one asked Jen about her mum. No one said Sally's name. Old friends avoided Jen because they didn't know what to say. And so, they said nothing. It was like Jen's mum had died a second time. Her dad resumed his travel, the house emptied, her grandmother did her best. After six months, the headmistress called Jen into her office.

'Are you all right?' she said.

'Yes . . .' said Jen, fearing she might be taken away from her remaining family if she told the truth.

'Very well.'

When your parents die, they move in with you. That was it. Jen didn't just lose her mum. She lost everything else too.

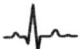

I have two wonderful daughters. Evie is the eldest – hard-working, studious, moody and slams her door. She loves reading and history and getting good grades. Dad is always embarrassing, and the very suggestion of a solution or idea means that it is the wrong suggestion or idea. And then there's Mimi – three years younger, red-haired and crazy. As a toddler, she would often lose her shit over something seemingly as inconsequential as not being allowed to eat her breakfast cereal with an ice cream scoop. She hasn't changed. And so, when Mimi made friends with a new girl at school called Catrin, who also had red hair, we knew we were in trouble.

We quickly realised that our small village lives had already crossed with Catrin's family. I had trained at the gym with Catrin's mum, and my wife went to exercise classes with her dad. We had many mutual friends and our lives had criss-crossed without meeting. We also remembered that Catrin's mum Charlotte had died from a brain tumour when Catrin was just ten.

Even though my days working in the Intensive Care Unit are spent walking hand in hand with death, we fell into the same trap as Jen's friend when Catrin first came to our house. We avoided topics that included 'mums' and at Christmas or on birthdays we steered towards the fun and away from the loss. But Catrin knew better. She was braver than us. When baking, she would say 'Mum used to love making these' or 'my mum had red hair too, we called her a lion'. And so we took her lead and leaned into it. We started asking to see photos of her mum and talking about her on Mother's Day. We lit a candle for Charlotte at a church service to remember people who had died. We allowed her to be remembered for what she was, 'an inspirational and unfalteringly brave woman, kind and selfless with an eternal smile', as described by her husband Dafydd and eldest daughter Freya. But it wasn't all doom and gloom either. Eulogies that are written about people often exclude the awkward bits, the quirks or the cracks. But we must remember that, as Leonard Cohen said, 'cracks let the light in'. So when our family went to a fundraising gym workout to support Brain Tumour Research, friends reminisced how Charlotte's funeral was as much a celebration of the cracks as well as the light that made her an incredible woman, with as many laughs as there were tears.

It has been said that you die twice – once when your body dies, and the next when people stop saying your name. During that charity event, more than a hundred people worked through punishing exercises in pairs while Charlotte's favourite music played. Dafydd cooked with Freya, while Catrin and my daughter Mimi paired up. And this was all in the name of Charlotte – literally – as each new exercise in sequence spelled out her name in bold letters for everyone to remember. Charlotte will only die once thanks to those who did, and always will, love her and keep saying her name.

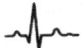

As if school wasn't hard enough for Jen, her own symptoms then started. Although she was sporty, enjoying hockey, tennis and squash, cross-country runs became impossible for Jen. She just couldn't run the distance. After being shouted at by her PE teacher for stopping during one lesson, Jen noticed the hill on the way home from school felt steeper. From fourteen, Jen would stop to tie her shoes halfway up rather than tell her friends that she felt out of breath.

But at least when Jen got home, there was always a welcome. Not a human welcome, but from her animal friends that filled the house – geckos, toads, rats and her elderly cat Sam.

'Sam was my best friend, my confidant and rock,' Jen told me. 'He would keep me company when my dad was away, always sleeping on my bed.'

And so, when Sam stopped drinking, Jen carried him to the vet, retracing the journey towards the hospital where her mum had died. Minutes later she left empty-handed. Like her mum, Sam had gone into a building never to come out. This experience led Jen to study animal care at agricultural college before applying to Aberystwyth University.

After arriving at university, Jen's nemesis was not the difficulty of the work nor the Welsh pronunciations, but the steep hill leading to her lecture theatre. Tying her shoelace was no longer enough, so Jen carried a digital camera, stopping to take photos during the breathless climb. She first rested halfway, then a quarter of the way a month later, then every 50 metres by Christmas. Jen's breathing was getting progressively worse and deep down she knew she had the same problem as her mum. She started staying at the top of the hill all day, not returning to her flat and not going out with friends to avoid any long walks home. Jen lost her friends once again.

Without family to fall back on and her dad not around, Jen was virtually adopted by her boyfriend's family, her 'angels', who lived on a working farm close by. By nineteen, after dropping out of university due to her health, Jen was given the diagnosis she knew all along and hoped wouldn't be true. She had severe heart failure just like her mum. She needed a transplant just like her mum. And Jen thought that she would die just like her mum.

Incredibly, this realisation did not define her. It did not change her. It didn't make her sad or angry or different. Jen rode quad bikes around the farm, worked outdoors as a labourer, went skiing on dry slopes. She was slow, had to stop frequently, but this was just life for Jen. And she wanted to grasp at every second of life to live it now, not then.

A Heart in a Jar

She struggled, but her friends now knew that she was ill. And so they understood. They adapted.

Having knowledge and talking about her illness, but not being her illness, almost made Jen normal. In fact, no, not normal – but supernormal. Jen even went back to university.

'It was just stuff to go through,' said Jen. 'It is much easier when it is happening to you. You have little control so why not go along for the ride? Life is life. All I wanted was to live life while I had one. Stopping would mean I had died while still being alive.'

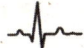

How can we keep on keeping on when all is falling down around us?

> The Sultan asked Solomon for a Signet motto, that should hold good for Adversity or Prosperity. Solomon gave him, 'This also shall pass away.'
>
> 'Solomon's Seal'
> by Edward FitzGerald, 1852

While the world around us can feel like a meticulously composed symphony, we find ourselves amid an impromptu jazz solo, grappling with the unexpected notes of life. Such was the case for renowned Portuguese pianist Maria João Pires, whose story is a tiny fragment of chaos compared with Jen but still resonates with the resilience, adaptability and the value of support in our most trying moments. Like Jen, she just had to see her mistake as 'stuff to go through' as there were no other options.

On a crisp autumn evening, Maria sat behind the grand piano at the heart of a bustling Royal Concertgebouw in Amsterdam. The 2,000-strong audience had taken their seats for an open rehearsal. Regarded as a leading interpreter of eighteenth-century music, Maria was the perfect replacement for a performance of Mozart's *Piano Concerto No. 20 in D minor* after another artist had to drop out. In a video taken of the event, you can almost see the weight of anticipation pressing down upon her shoulders as the crowd fidgeted in their seats. With 4,000 eyes fixed upon her, Maria floated her fingers above the piano's keys, ready to delve into the complexities of the concerto. As the orchestra's first notes filled the air, Maria's world came to a sudden, jarring halt.

In a split second, Maria's meticulously laid plans crumbled. The concerto she had expected to play was 'K.466' after mishearing 'K.488' during a phone call late the evening before. Panic, sharp and unyielding, threatened to engulf her. Yet, in the midst of this turmoil, the encouraging glance of the conductor, akin to a lighthouse in a tempestuous sea, offered her a glimmer of hope. Like Jen's adopted supporters, there was hope in others and well as in herself.

Drawing a deep breath, Maria closed her eyes, allowing the cold shower of fear to pass. With the conductor's supportive gaze, he mouthed words of support. She mouthed back, 'I'll do what I can do.' Maria embarked on an emotional journey through the notes of a piece she had not played in ten months. Each note a step in the dark.

When the concerto was first performed in 1785 many thought the whole thing was a big mistake. Audiences at the time saw concertos as pure entertainment. So when Mozart wrote a new concerto in a minor key, with aching anxiety and shivers of fear, he had taken a major risk. The picky Viennese nobility, on whose financial support Mozart depended, could have hated it. Instead, by breaking the rules, Mozart transformed the piano concerto for ever from joyful entertainment into a vehicle for deep emotional reflection.

So it was for Maria. She navigated the unexpected concerto, her music transcended mere notes on a page. It became a narrative of resilience, a melody of adapting on the fly – a harmonious blend of plans, mistakes and spontaneous recovery. The concert hall, once a daunting arena of expectation, transformed into a sanctuary of shared human experience, echoing with the warmth of collective support and understanding.

The standing ovation that greeted Maria's final note was not just in admiration of her musical talent but in recognition of her remarkable journey from panic to poise. It was a celebration of her ability to dance in the rain, to turn a potentially paralysing mistake into a powerful, unplanned masterpiece.

Life, in its essence, is an improvisation. Our plans may

serve as a guide, but it's our ability to adapt, supported by the belief and encouragement of those around us, that shapes our most defining moments. In embracing our vulnerabilities and the unforeseen challenges that come our way, we uncover the strength to transform setbacks into opportunities for growth and learning. In many ways, everything happens to everyone. We will all have terrible and wonderful things happen to us.

As the applause faded, Maria's journey through the uncharted waters of Mozart's D minor concerto stood as a testament to the beauty of mistakes and the transformative power of support. It was a vivid reminder that, in the grand concerto of life, it's not the notes we intended to play but how we play the unexpected ones that define our most memorable performances.

Perhaps jazz drummer E. W. Wainwright sums it up best, saying, 'A mistake is the most beautiful thing in the world. It is the only way you can get to some place you've never been before. I try to make as many as I can. Making a mistake is the only way that you can grow.'

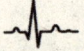

Jen didn't know if she would live long enough to have a transplant. When at university she carried a bulky pager everywhere she went. During her final exams, the device flashed every few seconds while on the invigilator's desk. In the summer, the time Jen had spent taking photos to slow down her walking led to her working as a wedding photographer. Soon, her images of wildlife captured in the New Forest hung on the walls of exhibition halls and art shops.

And it was during her search for wild deer to photograph that her life changed. Jen drove her fox-red Land Rover, dressed in wellington boots and waterproofs as Jack Johnson's latest album *In Between Dreams* spilled out from the open windows. The melody of his song 'Sitting, Waiting, Wishing' was interrupted by the pager's high-pitched beeping. A three-point turn in the middle of a country road took Jen back to her surrogate family's farm as the Sunday roast was arriving on the kitchen table. A bag was hastily packed as an ambulance arrived to take Jen to her new life.

Jen was determined to make the most of the journey to the hospital. It could have been her last. 'If I die, this is how I want people to remember me' she told the paramedics as she sang loudly along to the radio sat in the front of the ambulance on the one-and-a-half-hour drive on blue lights the whole way. They bounced on and off the hard shoulder, parting lanes of cars like the Red Sea.

'I expected to die like my mum,' she told me.

Does it surprise you that Jen was so happy yet so ill? Was she just really brave? Would you sing along to the radio or turn inward? In today's world of microaggressions and gaslighting, we should remember how amazingly resilient humans can be. Remember how strong you are.

Imagine if tomorrow you win the lottery. Within twenty-four hours, £10 million lands in your bank account. Life is transformed overnight. Now, contrast your new-found fortune with your next-door neighbour's imaginary change in fortune. A tragic accident leads to their right leg being amputated. Within twenty-four hours, their life too is transformed. At first glance, your stroke of luck and their misfortune appear at opposite ends of a happiness spectrum. Yet, when researchers probed deeper in the '70s study 'Lottery Winners and Accident Victims: Is Happiness Relative?', their findings challenged conventional wisdom about happiness and contentment.

The initial euphoria your experience as a new millionaire will gradually fade, a phenomenon psychologists call the hedonic treadmill. Your new wealth brings its own stresses and complexities, diluting the pure joy anticipated. Meanwhile, your neighbour, confronted with a reality that could easily engender despair, will likely embark on a journey of adaptation. They may find a deep spring of resilience and contentment that defies expectations. They are stronger than they think. We all are.

The critical lesson here, born from years of detailed research findings, is the human capacity for adaptation. Our happiness set-point, much like our ability to cope with stress, is remarkably malleable. We discover that external circumstances, whether fortuitous or catastrophic, only partially dictate our sense of well-being.

The study showed that happiness exists outside many objective life circumstances. Attitude and perspective colour experiences as much as actual events. These so-called contrast effects mean events seldom have set values – 1 point bad or

10 points good. Instead, we compare one thing to another. Meaning that winning the lottery is so good, it can even make other good things in life less enjoyable. Humans also quickly become habituated. After time, one leg doesn't seem so bad, and £10 million doesn't seem as good.

This tale underscores the importance of internal resources – grit, gratitude, perspective – in navigating life's vicissitudes. It's not the absence of stress that defines our well-being but our response to it. Understanding the complex interplay between luck, choice and resilience offers a richer blueprint for pursuing happiness.

In the end, happiness or meaning is less about what happens to us and more about how we interpret and respond to those events to an extent. It's a reminder that, in the quest for well-being, winning the lottery is not the important bit, rather it's having resilience, adaptability and perspective when we find out that we have lost.

Jen expected to die like her mum. So when she woke up after her transplant her words were simple. 'I did it. I'm alive!' She held up both thumbs and did a little happy dance. After just sixteen days in hospital, most of Jen went home. Her old heart stayed behind.

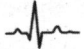

Every heart transplant procedure is remarkable, but the one I saw was nothing short of awesome, in the original meaning of the word. Sharareh Ahmadzadeh was a 28-year-old teacher who had travelled the world over seven years. While in Croatia, her last country before returning home to Australia, Sharareh became unwell with breathing difficulties put down to a simple common cold. But within weeks of being back at home, she was diagnosed with cardiomyopathy, or heart failure. Unlike Jen's inherited condition, Sharareh's heart problem was likely caused by a virus. Three weeks after her 'common cold', Sharareh was on the urgent heart transplant list.

Despite the fantastic people, facilities and healthcare system in Western Australia where Sharareh lived, there is a big problem – it is big. Really big. Western Australia is ten times the size of the UK yet with only the population of Wales. And while this makes it an awe-inspiring region to live and travel, Western Australia is terribly designed if you need a heart transplant.

When removed from the body, any organ has only a limited shelf life despite being put on ice. Hearts are particularly sensitive to being detached from their original owners and transporting them from any further away than Adelaide (around three and a half hours' flight time) would be too far. So the likelihood of finding a good match for Sharareh within that tight time and geographical window was very small. That's where a box comes into play – not any old cardboard box but a $500,000 TransMedics Organ Care System box. This technology allows patients in Perth like Sharareh to receive healthy hearts from places as far away as Sydney or even New Zealand.

Watching a glistening red heart arrive in a transparent

box, squeezing, twisting and beating without anyone near it, was one of the highlights of my time working in the cutting-edge transplant unit in Perth.

After a heart is carefully removed from a donor, it is placed in the TransMedics' sterile chamber and connected to a sophisticated perfusion circuit. This supplies the heart with a warm, oxygenated, nutrient-rich blood solution, maintaining conditions similar to those inside the human body. The heart is continuously monitored for function and viability, with real-time data on parameters such as temperature, pressure and flow rate. Unlike traditional cold storage, which limits transport time to a few hours, the TransMedics system can keep the heart viable for up to eight hours. This extended preservation time allows for longer transportation distances, ensuring that the organ remains healthy and functional until it reaches the recipient, thereby increasing the success rate of transplants and expanding the donor pool significantly.

After an eight-hour operation, Sharareh became the first person in the southern hemisphere to benefit from this technology, pioneered locally by surgeon Dr Robert Larbalestier. Sharareh has since returned to doing what she loves – working as a teacher, travelling and even running the 7.5-mile City to Surf charity race from Perth's city centre to its ink-blue sea.

The 'heart in a box' is more than just a device; it is a symbol of hope and progress. It ensures that distance is no longer a barrier to life-saving transplants. It allows an ever-widening moral circle, where empathy and ethical responsibility should extend to all humans (and many non-human animals), irrespective of location. The heart in a box reinforces the philosopher Peter Singer's vision of a more interconnected and compassionate world. The ability to share organs across great distances underscores global co-operation and mutual aid, demonstrating how modern innovations can bring us closer to realising a universally altruistic society. Sometimes, we need to think both inside and outside the box.

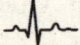

Eight years later, Jen was living an amplified life. Every day was a 'yes day', from climbing the tallest mountain in Wales, Yr Wyddfa, with her dog Bramley, to finding a job she loved helping young people excluded from school to learn outdoors. Then she fell in love. First dates are always tricky, but Jen's tattoo on her left wrist of a heart in a jar was an obvious icebreaker. When her date inevitably asked about it, Jen's answer would often result in no second date. People can be afraid to fall for someone with a complex health story. But when she met Tom, a healthcare software engineer, he just thought it was cool.

And eight years later, Jen read a letter that changed the lives of two families. During a routine hospital appointment, Jen's heart specialist handed her a white envelope. Inside was a handwritten letter from the family of a person whose death had given Jen life. It is their heart that now beats inside her chest. Unlike others in this book, Jen will never be able to thank that person who saved her life.

But she remembers them everyday thanks to her heart in a jar tattoo. Waking up next to her now husband Tom, Jen opens her eyes every morning to what is written below the colourful ink heart – 'vitam vive', or live life. Simple. Yet we simply forget. We always exist on the brink of the unknown, the imperfect. Wait for absolute security before seeking knowledge or beauty or adventure, then you will wait for ever.

I asked Jen what advice she can give people reading this who have only known life and not death. She looked up and smiled. She recounted a time when someone shouted at her for parking in a disabled parking space during one of her lowest times. Being young she was seemingly healthy from the outside.

'Be nice. Be kind. You never know what people are going through. But also, live life. Today. Use those plates you are keeping for a special occasion. Wear that special ball dress covered in plastic wrapping. In case that special day never comes.'

And eight years later, Jen was standing in the middle of a glass-clad, white-light-bright museum in London. She spent countless days looking at artefacts in display cabinets as a child due to her dad's work collecting specimens from around the world. But this specimen was different. It was familiar yet Jen had never seen it before. It gave her life and yet also took her life away. A narrow single spotlight shone down from above on to a small glass box. The room was drained of colour apart from this pink and purple structure. Suspended in clear liquid sugar was Jen's old heart.

How better to reflect on this life than to look at what gave you life in the first place. You don't have to have a transplant to do that. Look at your parents or the stars in the sky.

'Even when I am not here, when I die, my heart will tell my story to others. Perhaps it will make them think about their own life a little differently.'

7

Go Nuts

Alex, twenty-five years old
Cause of death: Allergy
Cause of life: Music is the operating system for the soul

It was the most delicious bowl of cornflakes Alex had ever eaten. Sadly, they weren't just cornflakes. Instead, the most allergic boy in Britain had eaten a large serving of cereal covered in tiny crunchy nuts. And then he died.

I first met Alex, unconscious and fighting for his life, shortly after I had returned from a book festival in Bali. There I had become vegetarian through writing my book *One Medicine*, which explores the extraordinary lives of animals. My protein sources changed overnight from chickens and cows to cashews and chestnuts. Nuts had become my friend but not for Alex, who had reacted dangerously to nuts, eggs and even peas since he was a baby. After spending months in London's Great Ormond Street Hospital as a child, Alex returned home to a new, adapted life. In school, Alex sat on a dedicated table with just one 'nut free' friend. Before football matches, he needed inhalers to fight off asthma attacks that would flare up each biting British winter. And birthday parties never ended with a slice of cake. Following in the footsteps of his Welsh great-grandad Mansel Treharne Thomas, one of the most influential musicians of his generation, Alex played the euphonium despite it making his face go red alongside the eczema related to his allergies.

Alex's parents, both in the police force, divorced when he was ten. Alex kept a strong relationship with both his mum and dad thanks to the time he spent with them at football matches, holidays abroad and long, lazy Sunday lunches with his sister at their Wiltshire childhood home. It was during one of these trips with his dad that Alex had a cardiac arrest after eating breakfast at a hotel in Cardiff.

Alex and his dad were visiting my home city of Cardiff to watch London-born singer-songwriter Freya Ridings. Her chilled-out piano music performed in Wales's St David's Hall was a perfect vibe for the cosy winter night with father and son. With last night's songs still playing in his head, Alex wandered around the hotel breakfast buffet, avoiding the foods he knew would spell trouble. The cornflakes he chose were the nicest bowl of cereal Alex had ever eaten – probably because it was the first time he had ever eaten the unlabelled nut-based crunchy cereal. The trouble is they tasted too good. As Alex was about to return for a second helping, he felt terribly sick, rushing up the three flights of stairs to his room on the top floor of the hotel. Realising what had happened, Alex tried to make himself sick before swallowing a handful of his anti-allergy tablets then punching his EpiPen through his jeans into his left thigh. By the time his dad got back to the room, Alex was bright red and struggling to breathe. 'It felt like Darth Vader had taken over my lungs,' Alex told me when we were reunited three years later. Alex collapsed to the floor as the medical team arrived, whispering to his dad, 'I think this is it.'

Chatting to Alex three years after he thought that was it, he showed me a blurred photo of his lifeless body lying on the hotel floor taken by his dad as the medical team saved his life. Alex was barely recognisable – his blotchy red skin replaced by a now pale, healthy complexion, a ripped T-shirt with defibrillator pads stuck to his skin replaced by a neat blue ironed fleece. Alex's surroundings were radically different too – gone was the hotel floor scattered with medical equipment and blurred paramedics sweating doing CPR. Instead, Alex spoke to me from a calm, tidy room at his sister's house with a black piano just visible in the background. Thankfully, public and commercial awareness of severe allergies has also moved on. Sadly, this came too late for 15-year-old Natasha Ednan-Laperouse, who tragically died in 2016 as she flew over the River Seine to Nice after eating an unlabelled sandwich containing sesame seeds.

The medical team who saved Alex needed to do three

A SECOND ACT

rounds of CPR, pumping in fluids, adrenaline and other drugs to put him safely on to a portable life support machine right there in the hotel room. Their next challenge was getting Alex to my hospital. Although only a few miles away horizontally, Alex was trapped in a cramped top-floor hotel room without a lift, the only escape through winding steps down narrow corridors. It took the fire service three hours to safely winch him from the top-floor window while still unconscious on a life support machine.

I met Alex after this tortuous journey in the resuscitation bay of the emergency department. It had already been a tough shift, too many patients with not enough beds. But as the emergency buzzer screeched out, the report came through of a young patient in cardiac arrest from a severe allergy. All the staff suddenly found an extra dose of energy from somewhere. After bursting through the doors, it was clear that the large bowl of cereal was still causing chaos inside Alex. Although our drugs were keeping him alive, the best action is always to fix the root cause in patients who are critically ill. So we sucked out as much of the congealed food as we could using tubes into Alex's stomach. But the thick mush wouldn't come up our pipes. So instead, we put down cameras like the ones used to unblock water-pipes and sucked up the remnants of the nutty cereal. We then put black charcoal into Alex's stomach to bind any remaining peanut proteins.

We used a powerful drug called aminophylline to open up the constricted passages in his lungs. You probably drink a similar drug yourself most mornings: caffeine is a naturally occurring phosphodiesterase inhibitor acting in a similar way to aminophylline, which can be used in rural locations without medical facilities to help treat tight lungs caused by allergies like Alex's or asthma. Chewing instant coffee may not be a pleasant experience but it can help save a life in people with severe asthma and no access to help. And all of this worked.

Over the next few hours, the amount of help Alex needed from our machines reduced, his face turned from Saturn red to salmon pink and his heart started squeezing once again. Within twelve hours, Alex was opening his eyes. Twelve hours later he was off the life support machine. And twelve hours later he was getting ready to go home. Just days after Alex died, he was back at work. And that is why I love caring for patients after cardiac arrests.

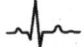

What's your favourite magic trick? Or top-rated miracle? The best scientific breakthrough? I would say 'to bring someone back from the dead'. Much of human history has been moulded by such extraordinary claims of resurrection yet every day, in every town, in every hospital, and in every ambulance, these so-called miracles occur. Not thanks to God but thanks to science. Thanks to our incremental acquisition of knowledge and thanks to everyday people like you doing something as simple as pressing on someone's chest. It is not always the right thing to do of course. When someone's heart stopping is simply the end result of another irreversible process, be it cancer or infection or heart disease, pressing on the heart won't work and wouldn't be right. But when a cardiac arrest happens suddenly for unknown or fixable reasons, CPR saves lives.

The week that Alex's heart stopped, the hospital where I work was leading one of the world's largest studies on caring for patients after a cardiac arrest. Studies like these are difficult to do, not least because patients are unable to give consent unlike other medical studies. After a cardiac arrest, people are often unconscious, many have brain injuries and although we could ask their family, these same people might have just done CPR on their son or daughter, mum or dad. These lifesavers are often unable to sleep, eat or drink afterwards yet alone synthesise the risks and benefits of a clinical trial on behalf of someone that they love who has just died.

Some say we just shouldn't do research in these situations. That it is unfair, unethical or not right. That instead we should just keep doing what we have always done. Yet critically ill patients, especially those suffering from cardiac arrest, are the most vulnerable to medical harms, the most in need of better treatments and actually the ones most in need of high-quality medical research. Out of 100 people who have a cardiac arrest outside of hospital, only ten of them will get to hospital alive. And from these ten people, five will die and three will survive but with severe brain injury meaning life will never be the same again.

Out of 100 people, just two will return to their second act like Alex. The 2 per cent club. And that is just not good enough. Thanks to large international trials like those co-ordinated by my colleagues, we are making progress in allowing more people to have a second act. We want more people like Alex.

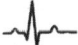

But there are other ways to save a life. To save many lives. Five years ago, I was lying down on a hard table with my trousers around my ankles, with two strangers holding my testicles while making small talk. As a 40-year-old with 2.5 children (two daughters and a dog), what better gift for my birthday than a vasectomy? The gift that hopefully stops giving was planned months before I turned forty. I thought I would be embarrassed after finding out a medical school friend does all the vasectomies in my local area. We had previously shared drinks and songs and anatomy books. I hoped he had remembered the anatomy but forgotten the songs. Thankfully, the considered environment, the preparation and the people made the whole experience easy and not awkward. The nurse who assisted him chatted as my friend cut into my scrotum. The sedative I was given even made the walk around the small, picturesque village where the clinic was, searching for my lift home, almost relaxing despite my unusual gait. It was like a scene from a zombie movie with around ten similarly aged men limping around slightly disorientated in jogging bottoms.

A SECOND ACT

The hard bit actually came sixteen weeks later when I needed to provide a sample. Although I understand why a semen sample had to be delivered within an hour of production, this was tricky. Especially as I live more than an hour away from the hospital. I faced a stark choice between speeding or getting caught in a compromising position in my own hospital office. Having navigated this first challenge (I'll leave my *modus operandi* to your imagination), I proceeded to the sample drop-off area clutching my cargo with five minutes to spare. Given that even beer bottles are wrapped in brown paper, it seemed unfair that the giant sample packaging was made from the world's most perfectly transparent material. What should have been a short walk down a corridor turned into a nightmare of bumping into colleagues like a wedding-greeting ceremony. Aware that the hour was nearly up, I had to lie and say I was delivering an important sample to the lab for a patient.

'Oh, I'm going that way, I'll take it for you,' said a helpful colleague reaching out to take the bag. Perhaps they noticed the giant oversized red capital letters spelling 'SEMEN' on the side as they accepted my lame excuse and walked on. With just two minutes to go, I arrived at my destination only to see a queue of guilty looking men all with identical sample containers. Each would take it in turn to press the wall intercom that was answered in a booming voice, 'SAMPLE DROP OFF?'

The oversized sign above the intercom read 'Fertility Centre' just to avoid any remaining uncertainty from the colleagues I had just met who now filed past me like slow buses. Finally, my turn came. With seconds to go, the door was opened and I handed my sample to the nurse. Or in my case, the hospital chaplain who had unfortunately been walking through the same door just ahead of the nurse.

This experience taught me a number of things. First, always check who you are handing your semen to. Second, despite having lovely, marvellous people in healthcare, we need to pay as much attention to the systems as the somebodies working within them. Complaints are often directed at people, yet the root causes are frequently found in poor systems or processes, not humans. I now appreciate the power of small changes. An opaque bag, a letterbox, a quieter intercom would not dilute the science but may make my next meeting with the hospital chaplain easier.

An email came out of the blue the evening after I was recovering from my vasectomy asking me to become an ambassador for the bereavement charity 2Wish. It was an invitation to attend their 'Little Ball of Hope'. It was the only little ball of hope I had left after my vasectomy so I immediately said yes.

2Wish support the friends and families of young people who have died, providing rooms for bad news to be broken, memory boxes that allow handprints and hair cuttings, and counselling in the days, weeks, months and years that follow when someone you love has died.

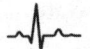

A SECOND ACT

I used to think I knew how to save a life. I've worked as a doctor for over twenty years, in intensive care as a consultant now for nearly ten. And the reason I chose that speciality wasn't the fancy machines, or the expensive drugs and certainly not long night shifts. It was because of a patient. It was because of one patient. He was called Chris.

Chris was a 17-year-old student, his life at his feet. Chris loved travel and music. He loved life. When Chris went on a school trip to Kenya something worried his parents, who tied a small piece of red wool to the roof rack of their car as they drove Chris to the airport. His dad told him that they would only untie that red wool when Chris returned home safely.

He never would. Because shortly after climbing Mount Kenya, Chris developed a temperature. This turned into a chest infection needing Chris to go to the local hospital. He became critically ill with sepsis and six weeks later was flown to Cardiff still attached to a life support machine. That was when I met Chris and his family.

It was the day after his eighteenth birthday party, held in the ICU, the day after he struggled to blow out the candles on his cake, that we told Chris' parents that he had died. We sat in the rubble with them. But there was nothing we could do. I remember everything about that day and visiting Chris's parents a decade later, so did they. They remember the relatives' room that was not fit for purpose, the peeling paint on the walls. They remember the specks of blood on the shoes of the staff. And they remember leaving the hospital with just a bag of Chris's clothes and a box of half-melted birthday candles. The red wool is still on their car today.

And so it was because of Chris that I decided to do intensive care medicine. I wanted to be able to answer the questions his parents had asked that day. Questions that many people ask when someone dies.

'Why did they die and yet others survive?'

'What more could have been done to save them?'

I spent decades trying to answer those two questions. Trying to save Chris's life again. I did research into sepsis, wrote books to explain things to the public. But I had forgotten about the third question that Chris's parents had asked. Perhaps I hadn't forgotten, perhaps I just didn't want to think about it because it was too hard. The third question his parents asked as they left the hospital was simple:

'What do we do now?'

And I had absolutely no idea. In my focus on saving Chris's life, I had forgotten about the other lives left behind. And I realised this as I read the invitation to the Little Ball of Hope.

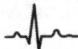

How can you save a life?

Well, you can't save a life using machines, or expensive drugs, or doing night shifts like me. But you can save lives by being there for people left behind in the wake of loss. By saying the names of those who have died like my daughter's friend's mum, Charlotte. And by just reading this book you are helping. I have committed to giving 10 per cent of profits from this book directly to 2Wish so that even when I cannot save a young person's life in ICU, those who remain can continue theirs. You are giving them practical support, a room where the paint is not peeling. You are giving them a memory box to take with them to remember those who have died that isn't a box of melted candles or a carrier bag of clothes. And you are giving them psychological support immediately after sitting in the rubble and years later. And so now, when I break the worst news to families as I do every day in the Intensive Care Unit, I can at least answer one of Chris's parents' questions – 'What do we do now?' You ask for help from organisations like 2Wish.

And for that I thank you. Thank you all. Thank you for supporting this cause. And I say this not only on behalf of those left behind, which one day could be you or I, but I thank you on behalf of healthcare staff like me. We all have what can be called 'those we carry'. Patients and families that we cannot forget even if we try. We see their shadows around corners on long night shifts, or at events like that Little Ball of Hope that I attended. That night, among the glittering ballgowns and manicured hair, I could see Chris sitting in my empty seat next to my wife as I spoke on stage. I saw others dotted around the room. And carrying these people can make you tired. But knowing that there is someone there to share that load, to offer them the support they need, makes the speech I gave not a sad one, but a happy one. Because those others I could see around the room had been supported by charities like 2Wish. I could see the people left behind who have had their lives saved, not by machines, or drugs, or doctors like me. But by others being there to support them.

At the end of that speech at the ball, I included words of wisdom from the Welsh language about these 4,000 weeks we have on Earth that we call life. I had asked an old childhood friend of mine for advice. Huw grew up in a busy, big, crazy household, always filled with music, people, family and his grandmother, or Mamgu as she was known in Welsh. Huw is a talented Welsh musician, poet and linguist. He first suggested *'yf dy gawl cyn oero'*, meaning 'eat your soup before it gets cold'. It was a perfect sentiment but as I was speaking during starters, I was actively making the soup go cold. So he instead settled on something said by St David, the patron saint of Wales and whom the concert hall Alex had visited was named after. As he died, Dewi Sant whispered:

'Gwnewch y pethau bychain mewn bywyd.'

'Do the little things in life.'

He wasn't talking about my vasectomy. He was talking about the little big things that really do matter. And who better to tell us about some of these little things than Huw's Mamgu, who died at the age of ninety-nine. Huw told me about his 'Mamgu's lessons for a happy life', which were:

A SECOND ACT

Cook for people
Keep some things for best
Remember your friends' birthdays
Write letters and cards to strangers
Visit those who can no longer visit you
Look through old cards, letters and photographs every
   year
Always keep a chair outside to enjoy the evening sun
Eat your soup before it gets cold

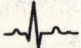

We return to Alex, whose body was back to normal but his mind was not.

'It was a struggle,' he told me. 'I should have been so happy but I was not. I just kept asking why? Why me? Why did I survive? Why am I alive?'

Struggling when amazing, rare or fortunate things happen is seen in corner cases of life – extreme situations that are hard to anticipate in advance. This existential experience has been described by people who have also needed a type of life support machine to stay alive like Alex, only not due to disease. Instead, they need specialised equipment to supply oxygen when they enter not a hospital but outer space. But why on Earth should space travel make you question life? And what can the experiences of astronauts tell us about life and death? How can they help Alex explain how he felt?

When Yuri Gagarin became the first human to leave our atmosphere, as breathtaking as the journey was out into space, it was the return trip to our little blue dot we all call home that was life-changing. Although psychologists worried that he might develop 'space madness' while in orbit, they didn't predict the so-called 'overview effect' that would be described twenty-five years later.

It was the experience of seeing Earth from the outside, hanging free against the vastness of space, that led to a fundamental change in a Gagarin worldview. He described this long before the term 'overview effect' was coined, saying, 'Orbiting Earth in the spaceship, I saw how beautiful our planet is. Let us preserve and increase this beauty, not destroy it.'

The overview effect is a cognitive shift during spaceflight, often while viewing the Earth from outer space. This effect encompasses feelings of awe, a deep understanding of the interconnectedness of all life, and a renewed sense of responsibility for taking care of our planet. Their narratives often touch on themes of unity, scale and the fragility of life – elements that dramatically widen their perspective and, occasionally, alter their approach to life upon return.

But there is an astronaut even more famous than Gagarin who can explain the links between the overview effect and survivors of cardiac arrest like Alex. They can also give us hope that we can get through tough times in our own lives.

When I say a more famous astronaut, I have stretched the truth a little. Because even though William Shatner has gone into space many hundreds of times more than Gagarin, on board his fictional starship *Enterprise*, it was not until

2023, aged ninety, when Shatner did it for real. After stepping off Amazon founder Jeff Bezos's commercial spaceship *New Shepard*, he said, 'I was crying. I didn't know what I was crying about. I had to go off some place and sit down and think, what's the matter with me? And I realised I was in grief.'

Similarly, individuals like Alex, who experience near-death situations such as cardiac arrests, often face a comparable profound shift. A grief of sorts. Loss of his former self or worldview. Grateful to be alive. But unsure what this life is now all about or ever was. After his anaphylactic shock, Alex's return from the brink was not just a physical recovery but also an intense psychological journey. Survivors often report feelings of disorientation, depression, or a deep existential searching akin to what astronauts like Shatner experienced after returning to Earth. This emotional turmoil is not the madness that worried space psychologists, but more a crisis of meaning and identity. In fact, it is the sanest feeling of all – what is this life really all about?

Like many people who survive the unsurvivable and arrive in a second act, rather than feeling ecstatic they can feel sad. Sad because they realise how precious life is, sad because suddenly they may look on their former life as lacking meaning, or sad because they see how cruel people can be on Earth despite the awe and beauty that surrounds us all.

Both astronauts and cardiac arrest survivors like Alex undergo a sudden expansion of perspective that forces a confrontation with existential realities. They face questions about purpose, the fragility of existence and their priorities in life. For Alex, his survival was not just a second chance at life but an invitation to re-evaluate what matters most. Just as astronauts may return with a new-found commitment to planetary stewardship or global unity, Alex found himself deeply contemplating how he wanted to use his regained life. He follows in a long tradition of our search for meaning.

So how do we combat this sense of nihilism, whether it is from space or from surviving death or just the everyday grind? Do we need to search for meaning in grand, worldly ways, big gestures and making an impact on the world?

For Alex, meaning eventually returned from deep down. Deep but different. Music had always been rooted in his heart but after his brass band folded, going back to the euphonium didn't feel right. Like a well-crafted plot of a novel, Alex returned to the music that surrounded him near his death. Freya Ridings' album that he listened to that winter night in Cardiff had been entirely written on piano. And as he returned to work, experienced the feelings of 'what now?', his old family piano called to him.

Tinkering on its keys led Alex from first learning to play his favourite songs to writing his own. And he loved it, partially because he was not good at it. Unlike his perfected brass tones, he would often hit a bum note or not hit a note at all. But that challenge, that exploration seemed to make it better. It also helped his hazy memory that he had struggled with since his heart stopped. Music is the operating system for the human soul.

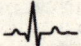

Sometimes life feels like one long competition. And perhaps you have already made it. Perhaps you have already won. You were born, you survived. You may have been a top student in school, or did better than your friends in exams. You may have played sport at a high level, aced your musical grades, or performed on stage in lead roles. Even if getting into work or university was a struggle, you overcame that. You persevered. You fought. You held on. Many of us start and remain competitive by nature.

But even when we 'make it', arrive in a job we always wanted or a place in life we have strived to, we sometimes engineer our own competition. For me, I stepped into roles in academia; for others they join the management escalator. We look to titles, committees and the conference stages to find meaning. Some doctors find competition in illnesses where only a cure equals a win, although this is a ghost that can't be held. This competitive nature isn't all bad, of course. We need driven, dedicated individuals who strive for their best as well as what's best for patients for those working in healthcare. But, just as we can't all be chosen to be the school team captain, there may remain a residue of discontent when we're left on the bench or playing for the third team.

So why not instead pour this competitiveness into something different, something pointless, or even something you're terrible at? Many of us do a version of this already. We may try to beat our 5K time at parkrun or plan a marathon before our fortieth birthday. We think back to our old personal bests and begrudgingly hold on with gritted, aged teeth. We may even discharge our competitive spirit at the weekly pub quiz or on a Sunday with a crossword. But I had always thought that these activities should be things we were already good at, or at least in pursuits we could become good at.

In a *Guardian* article headlined 'The joy of mediocrity', Kerri Duncan encourages us to find joy in what we're bad at. She writes, 'When I focus too much on getting better at something, it creates room for failure. I don't want to fail in my relaxation time.' This is a blissful contrast to the necessitated perfection in healthcare. Having even one moment when we're 'bad' at our job, by making what in other professions would be a very understandable and simple mistake, becomes a formal complaint or a patient's life. So allowing or even running towards incompetence in other parts of our lives may be a welcome change.

It's okay to join that choir even though you're a terrible singer, to paint if you can't paint, or to run if you can't run. You may never be able to chase away your inherently competitive nature that got you where you are, but that's okay as well. Perhaps after some time your voice will improve, your art will get better, or your 5K time will be shorter than your ward round. Pouring your competitive nature into something other than just your day job may allow mediocrity to improve your life, inside and outside your work, instead of only spelling failure.

And so, for Alex, if art was life, music was therapy. It shows that although this book encourages a YOLO (you only live once) approach to life, this doesn't mean splurging your savings, or making bad choices that you regret the next morning, or making massive waves of meaning in the globalised world. It means finding meaning in the small things. The little things that matter as Dewi Sant has told us. It means being open to new experiences whether it is swimming in the cold sea or learning to paint or playing the kazoo. Go on. Go nuts.

8

3 Billion Beats

Kai, thirty-eight years old
Cause of death: Too much life
Cause of life: More quit, less grit

The last time Kai's chest hurt this much, he had been giving CPR for hours. Now he was the one receiving it. Kai is a forty-something intensive care doctor just like me. But unlike me, he briefly died while staying in a rural cottage during a weekend reunion with old friends. Kai lived because his wife saved his life by doing CPR as their young children watched. And after reading this chapter, I hope you too will be able to save a life.

Growing up near Cambridge during the '80s, it was no surprise that Kai went into medicine. His mum was a nurse, his dad a leading equine vet, and his oldest sister a doctor. The small town of Newmarket was home to both his dad's work and the family of six, which included Kai and his three older sisters. Kai was a clever kid, enjoying athletics and rugby, but still needed to work hard to get the grades needed for medical school. At university, he really found his feet, enjoying the science, the camaraderie, and made friends for life. Friends he would meet again decades later in that Old Flour Mill cottage in the Peak District where his life changed.

There was one experience during Kai's second year as a doctor that made him want to pursue intensive care as a career. It was his first placement in the ICU and the start of a long run of night shifts. Within minutes of arriving at the evening handover, the emergency cardiac arrest alarm screamed out. For the next twelve hours it hardly stopped. It had been a very unusual night shift, far more cardiac arrests to manage than normal but the end of the shift was within sight. A colleague of mine often adapts the lyrics to the song 'Far Away' by the Levellers, saying, 'There's never been a night shift that lasts for ever.' While this is true, that last twenty minutes waiting for the fresh, daytime reinforcements to arrive feels like an eternity. And it was exactly twenty minutes before the end of Kai's night shift when the cardiac arrest alarm went off yet again.

It was the type of emergency that even the most skilled doctor dreads. After twenty years in medicine, it takes a lot to raise my resting heart rate but when the emergency buzzer's speaker calls out 'Cardiac arrest! Maternity suite!', mine still shoots sky-high. Kai realised that not one but two lives would be in his hands.

It was a difficult, emotional and traumatic cardiac arrest. The obstetricians needed to do an emergency Caesarean section while Kai continued to do CPR on Mum. Getting out and saving the baby was also the best way of saving Mum in this rare circumstance. After just minutes that felt like hours, the reassuring cries of a newborn screamed above the sounds and clamour of emergency machines beeping and people counting out aloud the rhythm of the CPR still being done on Mum by Kai. Baby survived. Mum died. And Kai needed to come back the next night and the night after that.

He still remembers how he felt in the days that followed. Not only was it traumatic emotionally, but he was also physically destroyed. His back, chest and arms seizing up during the next night as if he had been fighting for his own life not someone else's. 'Those shifts were exhausting, tough and fascinating,' he told me. 'I knew by the end of those night shifts that I definitely wanted to do intensive care.'

Like when I cared for Chris, the young 18-year-old student who died of sepsis, Kai's decision came soon after a tragic loss. There is something about the end, about death, that makes us strive to do more, to do better somehow. Walking towards difficulty is sometimes the easiest way to deal with it.

Admitting this is difficult. I've performed CPR hundreds of times and when I'm pressing on someone's chest, I don't think about the person beneath me, their life, or their death. I don't think about their family or what I'll say afterwards

A SECOND ACT

if they live, or if they die. I don't even think about myself. Or my own family. Or my dog. Instead, I think about everything. Everyone. This whole thing. This life.

I've been a doctor for twenty years, been busy for twenty years. I've had little time to stop and think. I've grown up, had children, lost children, loved, been loved, cried, laughed, and not yet died. I'm now the age that I used to think was old yet feel young. Younger gets older the older I am. And as I press up and down on someone's chest, these thoughts pour into my mind. Perhaps these two-minute cycles when I am doing CPR are the only times when I can truly reflect, be present.

And at the end of that pondering, another two minutes of my life and your life have passed. Another cycle of CPR will start, a colleague will take over from me and perhaps they too will stand there and wonder the same as I did. Perhaps, like me, they will eventually conclude that the meaning of life is less about finding answers, more about asking the question. Rather than ask, 'What is the meaning of life?', it is better to ask, 'How to bring meaning to a life?' Because meaning is not about being busy, or achieving everything, it's not about an 'inbox zero' or a bank balance. Meaning is not only hidden in grand moments like those when I'm doing CPR, but in the simple, everyday acts we all do every day. The unremarkable passing of the short time we have to question why.

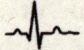

Life will never get easier. But you can get better at dealing with it. Working in the intensive care unit is to remain in a constant state of 'permacrisis'. The extraordinary becomes routine, the unexpected a daily occurrence. The structure of the day is imposed on the chaos to contain it within something more manageable. But it can still change at any second. A stable patient can die within minutes, someone critically ill facing their end can be saved by a needle or a knife seconds later. I can never get comfortable in a chair, never sit back without one eye on the next moment. On top of this, every routine 'day at the office' for me is the most important day in someone else's life. There are few jobs that demand this. Perhaps the vicar conducting yet another wedding feels the same pressure but doing a bad job wouldn't result in death.

This environment demands not only expertise but also a profound resilience and adaptability as we navigate the relentless tide of life-and-death situations. In such a high-stakes setting, strategies are essential to manage the continuous stress and maintain effective patient care. But these tactics are not useful only in the white-washed world of ICU. I think they would help in your life too.

One of the frameworks I use are checklists. These are not mere administrative tools but vital instruments that ensure nothing is overlooked in the midst of chaos. Checklists guide procedures, confirm critical steps and ensure consistency in patient care. They help mitigate human error, providing a cognitive safety net that allows staff to focus on the nuances of patient care rather than the mechanics of routine tasks. This systematic approach ensures that even under immense pressure, the standard of care remains uncompromised. Although I use checklists to safely insert tracheostomy tubes into patients' necks, I also use them to go on holiday. It makes that last-minute dash out of the door less stressful and has often prevented us from forgetting to turn off the heating or to bring a travel adapter. Checklists are for life, not just for tracheotomies.

Proactively planning and expecting disasters is another cornerstone of ICU preparedness. In an environment where rapid deterioration in a patient's condition is just around every corner, forward planning is crucial. We don't wait until the ventilator breaks or all power turns off to think about what to do next. These plans are meticulously developed, regularly updated, and rigorously drilled ahead of time. Simulations of cardiac arrests, multi-trauma admissions and other critical events prepare the team to act swiftly and cohesively. This anticipation and readiness for the worst-case scenarios fosters a culture of vigilance and proactive intervention, transforming potential crises into manageable situations. Life too has predictable disasters waiting for you. One day your car tyre will be flat, your only bank card will be declined, your parents will die. Doing some preparation, even if only cognitively, for these predictable surprises that will hit you on some idle Tuesday can really help.

Moreover, the emotional resilience developed in the ICU through continuous exposure to high-stress situations fosters in me a profound understanding of human fragility and strength. This perspective can cultivate empathy, patience and a deep appreciation for life's fleeting moments. It teaches me to value health, relationships and the time we have, recognising that every moment is precious and worth safeguarding. It teaches me that everything is relative. After caring daily for people at the brink of death, it makes that flat tyre or that declined bank card less scary. If I start whingeing to myself while running 5K as it starts hailing, I will think about the patients with spinal injuries who would give anything to be running with me in the cold and wet.

Putting yourself outside the boundaries of your work and your life could bring a similar perspective. Volunteer with those less fortunate than you. Read books about what life was like for your own family just a generation ago. Think back to your own past when life was tough and remember how far you have come. Channel your inner Mark Twain who said, 'I am an old man and have known a great many troubles, but most of them never happened.'

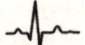

Ten years after Kai's chest was sore from trying to save that mum's life, doing CPR long enough to at least save her baby's life, he was in the final weeks of training to become an intensive care consultant. It had been a brutal few years with Covid, difficult exams to pass and research projects to complete as Kai also balanced the demands of being a dad to three young children. But there was a bench at the end of his long path. With his final placement nearly over, Kai looked forward to a long overdue reunion with friends, which had been rescheduled multiple times during the pandemic.

Taking turns driving to the Peak District, Kai and his family finally arrived after dark following his last ever night as a resident doctor. Coffee and loud music had helped them over the final miles and a cold beer and lifelong friends welcomed them through the doors of the Old Flour Mill cottage where they were all staying.

Good conversation and catching up on shared experiences got in the way of home cooking, meaning it was nearly midnight when they finally sat down to eat. The children formed a self-governing crèche, entertaining themselves with only the occasional need for a parent to step in with an emergency wet wipe. After the babies had been carried to their cots and the dishes piled next to the sink, Kai and his wife went to sleep with their walking boots left next to the cottage door ready for the planned morning hike.

Kai's youngest, three-month-old Dylan, woke for a feed just after 3 a.m. but was soon back asleep after Kai took on burping duties. As he held Dylan against his chest, Kai felt sweaty, sick and like he was about to die. He was.

After quickly handing the baby to his wife, Kai collapsed on the bed, fitted and hit his head on the thick wooden bedside table. It was thanks to what his wife did next that Kai's life was saved. Would you know what to do? Could you save a life?

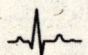

3 Billion Beats

Despite our fancy machines and expensive drugs in ICU, the most powerful tools to save a life when someone has a cardiac arrest are not mine, or in the hospital. You have them. You can save a life.

We all have the potential for 3 billion heartbeats during our lifetime. We all die many times each day, in the pauses between these 3 billion heartbeats. But every year, 30,000 people in the UK will suddenly collapse to the ground having suffered a cardiac arrest before they get there. Their heart will either have stopped beating completely like Kai's, started fibrillating (jittering) 200 times a minute, or will be unable to pump blood despite the electric circuits working correctly. Two out of ten of those people will survive, and one will have what we call a 'good neurological outcome'. That person will get back to work, live normally with their loved ones, do the things they love doing. And that is phenomenal. It is one of the medical conditions that always astounds me, where people go from being dead to fully alive once again. It feels like magic.

But it is also tragic. Because if bystander CPR was always given, thousands more lives could be saved: thousands more husbands back to their wives, daughters back to their dads, friends to have coffee together again. If you did CPR on someone you saw having a cardiac arrest, they would be twice as likely to survive and return home. Why wouldn't you?

Well, bystanders can feel scared, worrying they'll get something wrong or cause more harm. But if someone is already dead, there is no harm you can do. The chances of surviving are doubled by prompt CPR (and defibrillation), and because around 80 per cent of cardiac arrests happen in the home or the workplace, there is often someone close by who might be able to help. That person one day could be you.

Doing CPR is not complicated, you don't need to be a doctor or a nurse. I'm proud to say that my 11-year-old daughter Mimi learned how to do CPR at school because in Wales it's part of the curriculum. It's really one of the most important lessons schools can teach. Apart from simultaneous equations.

So, could you save a life? Yes. You need to make a choice whether this book will change not only your own future, but the life of someone else. Starting CPR early in cardiac arrest is critical to a good outcome. Even the fastest ambulance will not get to a patient and start CPR more quickly than you can. So let's do this. Please switch your phone on to silent, close the door and put down your drink.

First, put the hard heel of your right hand in the middle of your chest, between your nipples. Now put your other hand on top. Next, get ready to sing. Press your hands up and down on your chest in time with the start of every word while repeatedly singing aloud the Bee Gees' 1977 classic 'Stayin' Alive':

'Ah, ha, ha, ha, stayin' alive, stayin' alive Ah, ha, ha, ha, stayin' alive.'

In fact, any song at around 100 beats per minute will

work from 'I Will Survive' by Gloria Gaynor, Europe's 'The Final Countdown', or even Taylor Swift's 'You're Losing Me'.

Congratulations! You have just performed CPR in the correct position, pressing at just the right speed. Enrolling in a free CPR course will make you even better but from now on if you ever see an adult collapse, not breathing properly, and not showing any normal signs of life, you have the skills to help save them. Ensure the emergency services have been contacted, get down on your knees and simply do what we have learned. Keep your arms powerful and straight. Press down hard until you feel the chest move inwards. You cannot do more harm than good. You may save that person's life. Not doing it carries a much bigger harm – certain death. If you ever do save someone's life after reading this, please write and tell me. It will be the best letter I ever receive.

For even more structure, follow these steps:

Call for help
If someone has collapsed and is unresponsive, the first thing to do is call for help.

Try to wake them
Then try gently shaking their shoulders and calling their name to check for signs of consciousness.

Look and listen

Look and listen for signs of breathing – check if the chest is moving up and down at a normal rate. Has their breathing become shallow, irregular or stopped entirely? If the answer is yes to any of these, this is an emergency.

Call 999

Put your phone down and on speaker mode. The call handler will know if there is an automated external defibrillator (AED) nearby. If there is, send someone to get it. The emergency call handler will help by giving clear instructions on how to use one and how to give chest compressions.

Prepare to press

Put any hand on top of the other, interlock your fingers for stability. Then place the heel of your hands in the middle of the chest between the nipples. Start pumping firmly down, about twice every second in time to the Bee Gees' tune 'Stayin' Alive'. Don't worry if you don't know the song, being slightly slower or faster is much better than nothing.

Don't stop

You do need to press hard. It's natural to worry about hurting someone but good CPR often results in minor injuries like rib fractures. This means you are doing it right, not wrong. Doing CPR properly is tiring so rotate with others minimising the change over time until there are signs of life, or a defibrillator arrives. Don't stop.

How long should you carry on?
In short, until there are signs of life, or the paramedics arrive. When a natural pulse comes back, we call this 'return of spontaneous circulation'. Survival rates go down the longer this takes, but in stressful circumstances it's often hard to feel a pulse even for doctors. Seconds feel like minutes and minutes like hours.

Should I do 'the kiss of life'?
Unless you have been on an advanced course, the 'kiss of life' is no longer officially recommended for adults. The vast majority of cardiac arrests occur in adults aged 15–64, and are heart-related, so compression-only is the standard advice. Although I claimed in my last book, *One Medicine*, that kissing a frog really can save your life, so can kissing a French person who died 200 years ago. In fact, she is the most kissed person in the world.

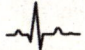

In the 1800s, death was not hidden away, rather it was even used as entertainment. The Paris morgue was known as the Theatre of Death, purposely located centrally on the banks of the Seine to collect people, help with identification and provide a spectacle with large viewing windows. It was the 'only free theatre in Paris'. Despite using cold water that dripped from the ceiling, without refrigeration the people on display would last only a few days. So a wax cast of the deceased's face would replace the body, allowing viewing and identification to continue.

One year, a girl around sixteen years old was found in the Seine, thought to have died by suicide. After a few days, as no one had claimed her body, her surprisingly calm smile was captured using a wax death mask. The viewing crowds that then gathered were so large that shops started selling souvenirs called *'L'In-connue de la Seine'*, 'The unknown woman of the Seine'. Despite her celebrity status, the young girl was never identified.

Fast forward to the 1940s, Norwegian toymaker Asmund Laerdal's son fell into a lake and nearly drowned. It was his dad's quick actions that saved him and subsequently inspired his toy-making skills to be adapted into the production of life-sized CPR training dolls. Making the mannequin bodies was simple enough, but when it came to the face, Laerdal remembered a calm, smiling death-mask that had hung on the wall of his family's home. It was *L'Inconnue de la Seine*. Using the newly developed post-war material called plastic, the unknown woman of the Seine became Laerdal's 'Resusci Anne'.

Anne has now been used to train more than 500 million people worldwide since 1960, including me, Kai and his wife, a GP. The Laerdal company estimates that more than 2 million lives have been saved thanks to the unknown woman as well as inspiring Michael Jackson's lyrics 'Annie, are you okay?'

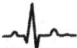

As Kai lies dead on his bed in the Old Flour Mill cottage, his wife saves his life. While Dylan lay next to Kai, his wife pressed on his chest. Like the maternal cardiac arrest that Kai managed early in his career, the future lives of both mum and baby could radically change. And Kai's chest hadn't felt this sore since then either. The two older children peered around the door frame, asking, 'Mummy, what are you doing?'

Dylan was placed on a single bed next to his dad, turned towards Kai's wife Seren as she did CPR perfectly. She screamed for help and friends soon burst into the bedroom. There were frantic calls to 999, made more difficult due to the weak phone signal and long Wi-Fi password. By the time an ambulance arrived, miraculously Kai was conscious. He tried to sit up and joked to his friends, 'If I did die, I can tell you now that there's nothing back there!'

No one laughed apart from Kai and his friend who was a surgeon. Like Kai, he experienced both sides of life and death many times a day at work, where humour was often the only way to keep going. But as soon as the chuckles stopped, Kai felt like he was going to die once again.

Kai's heart rate kept dropping to levels only seen in giant

creatures like the 200-tonne blue whale. Although beating just six times a minute is okay for a whale's heart, this is because so much blood is pumped out each time. Kai's human-sized heart would never get enough oxygen to his brain at such a low speed.

Despite realising his wife had just done CPR after feeling his sore chest, Kai wasn't afraid. He told me that the most scared he had ever been wasn't in that moment, but rather while working as a doctor on the top floor of an old hospital in Christchurch, New Zealand, ten years earlier. On Tuesday 22 February 2011 at 12.51 p.m. Christchurch was badly damaged by a magnitude 6.3 earthquake, killing 185 people and injuring several thousand. The earthquake's epicentre was just 6 miles south-east of Christchurch's main hospital. The shaking that Kai had felt at the top of that old building gave him a raw, primitive feel in his soul. 'I thought that was going to be it.' This actual scrape with death, however, felt different. 'I was dead, then I was alive again,' he said.

'It didn't really happen to me, it was my family and friends who went through it. Being dead isn't really that bad.'

Thinking about death can be hard. Like Kai, I'm not scared of being dead, but I am scared of dying. This is because death is a pain-free binary point in time just like the millions of years before you were alive. Dying is different, it is a process, non-binary, quantitative. You go through dying, you are there. We will all face both of those 'D words' at some point but many doctors, nurses, patients and families overdo a third 'D word' – denial.

In this longevity-obsessed world, we are becoming increasingly less able to countenance a natural death or to understand what truly matters in our final days. Instead, we channel our inner Dylan Thomas as we 'Rage, rage against the dying of the light'. The Intensive Care Unit where I work is a technical marvel. We have machines to temporarily replace your lungs, heart and kidneys. We have powerful drugs that pause your immune system, change your blood pressure and erase memories. And most importantly, we have staff with the skills to use them and mindset to care. After all, beds don't cure people, people cure people.

But for those who are already dying when they arrive in hospital, intensive care comes at a huge cost – both literally and figuratively. At a time when community and connection matter most, we too often default to high-tech but low touch. Moreover, misguided heroism on the part of medicine can mean whisking people away from those they love, from the homes and familiarity that they deserve. When the dying should be unencumbered, instead we insert more tubes than the average bagpipe. These well intentioned 'medical assaults' help all claim that we 'fought hard' and mean nobody is accused of 'giving up'. The discrepancy between what so many people want at the end and what they may receive is something we should all be raging about.

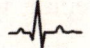

When it comes to death, making the diagnosis is emotionally draining, but has been central to the doctor's job for centuries. Surprisingly, British law does not provide an official definition of death. Instead, we rely on various guidelines, including one from the Academy of Medical Royal Colleges, which states:

> Death entails the irreversible loss of those essential characteristics which are necessary to the existence of a living human person and, thus, the definition of death should be regarded as the irreversible loss of the capacity for consciousness, combined with irreversible loss of the capacity to breathe.

When I am called to confirm death, I perform the same ritual each time. First, I talk to the dead. In intensive care, patients often have their eyes closed, either from sedation or illness. But I still talk to them, explaining my actions. We are often surprised when recovering patients recall fragments of their unconscious time. And so, for me, communication remains crucial even when extended beyond death, even when no response is expected.

I begin by saying hello and introducing myself. 'I'm feeling for your pulse,' I say. Placing my index and middle fingers on their neck, I feel for the characteristic tapping of the carotid artery. Simultaneously, I position my stethoscope on their chest, listening for the lub-dub sound of the heart valves. Then I wait – a long, silent, slow five minutes. I listen for silence, feeling for the presence of absence. No sound is heard, and no pulse is felt. This confirmation can be chilling. Your mind plays tricks as you feel your own pulse and hear your own heartbeat.

Next, I open the patient's eyes and shine my pen torch into the depths of their pupils, the black space between the front and back of the eyes. We all have this crack in our eyes, that's how the light gets in. In life, the pupils would constrict to a tiny speck of black, but in death, they remain large and dark, like windows no longer looking out. Finally, I press firmly on the bony ridge above the eye, saying softly, 'I'm sorry.' Nothing happens. The patient is dead.

Talking about death is much harder than its confirmation. I have around 200 difficult conversations every year, telling people that their husband, wife, brother, mother, dad, sister, friend, lover has died or will never be the same again. Each conversation, saying sorry, watching other people cry with hope and fear, takes a tiny piece of flint away from my core. All in the knowledge that one day that will be you. The timing is just as cruel. I've confirmed death on people's birthdays, wedding days, children's first birthdays. Days they are due to watch their favourite band, go on that big trip, ask someone to marry them.

The reactions of a family to bad news are equally as broad as the tragedies involved. People cry, scream, laugh, run away, thank us, understand, hit the wall and hit themselves, hit others. They beg us to be wrong, they deny death is actually possible, and even the atheist can plead to God for a miracle. These reactions are not right or wrong, they are just part of human grief and the sacrifice needed to make love possible.

Modern medicine is a marvel, but can be a curse, especially for frail, older people, and particularly those with terminal disease. Honest, direct, careful communication helps everyone understand that an end is approaching and is likely unavoidable. Being the doctor who is called in at the eleventh hour, there has often been a lot of obfuscation in the lead up. Communication has always been the most important procedure in medicine. I've moved beyond euphemisms and instead prescribe compassionate candour. Now clarity is important. I've borrowed a phrase from palliative care physician Dr Kathryn Mannix and often simply say, 'They are sick enough to die.'

Just as language surrounding the end is key, so too are the words when a patient has actually died. The power of disbelief grows in grief, making families interpret words in a way that is least painful. 'I'm afraid we have lost your mum', or 'Your dad is no longer with us', or 'Your son has gone to a better place' will be interpreted literally. 'Where have they gone?' comes the reply. Instead, I confront reality and say, 'I'm very sorry, but they have died.'

Not only are too many patients not getting what they deserve, it's also not happening where they want. For example, once upon a time, humans died at home, surrounded by family, friends, neighbours and pets. As the mortician Caitlin Doughty explains, 'Home was where the death was.' The wider community came together and spent the time – whether hours, days or weeks – making sense, finding courage, teaching and learning. Hands were held, tea was poured, cakes were baked and dogs were petted. Nowadays, dying hides in plain sight. It is institutionalised, technologically mediated, and obscured by monitors and Latin words. In hospitals, the tea, cake and pets are frequently banned, and family visitation is policed. I can still claim expertise because we know the pills and machines. But I'm happy to admit my amateur status when it comes to helping families make sense, connections and meaning. Dying should be nurtured by society, instead it has been hijacked by 'big medicine' or 'big death'.

The change was inevitable. In 1950, a forefather of critical care warned, 'At the beginning of ICU it is a problem to keep the patient alive, eventually it will be a problem to let them die.' It has taken courage to grow intensive care into a specialty that has saved countless lives. It will take the same candour to mature into a specialty that saves as many deaths.

For balance, it is important to understand that we have also institutionalised death because it can be traumatic when it happens at home. This is why more resource should be allocated to palliative care, keeping people in their communities and alongside friends. And despite his initial protestations, even Dylan Thomas came to realise this. In his poem 'Do Not Go Gentle into That Good Night', the early denial of his dad's death may have inspired 'rage', but even this firebrand eventually admits that 'wise men at their end know dark is right'. The trouble is that wise men and women may not be the ones doing the resuscitation – they may be the ones forced to receive it.

In her job as a GP caring for elderly, frail people in care homes, Seren would regularly have conversations about CPR. But after we have learned about these marvellous resuscitation techniques, one might wonder why doctors shouldn't try to save the lives of everyone having a cardiac arrest. How could a DNACPR (Do not attempt cardiopulmonary resuscitation) order ever be a moral choice?

There are two distinct scenarios in which cardiac arrest occurs. The first involves a patient who develops a primary problem with the heart or other organs, resulting in an unexpected cardiac arrest. This could be caused by a sudden heart attack, a clot in the lungs, or significant trauma. In these cases, we do everything humanly possible to 'fix' the underlying problem while performing CPR to buy us time. The lengths we will go to may even involve performing life-saving open-heart surgery at the side of the road, as one of my medical school colleagues in the Welsh air ambulance service did in 2017.

The second scenario is when a cardiac arrest occurs in a patient with a severe underlying disease that has reached its end stage. Patients with chronic heart disease, lung disease or terminal cancer will all die *with* a cardiac arrest. They do not die *from* a cardiac arrest; they die from their original disease. We all eventually die the same way: our heart stops. In these circumstances, the cardiac arrest signals that the underlying disease cannot be fixed. Pressing on the heart will only result in the loss of dignity for the patient and emotional distress for the medical team. There is nothing to fix, so any extra time CPR gives simply prolongs death rather than life.

Put in these terms, it's hard to understand why anyone would insist on having CPR during the twilight of their life. If asked, most people don't. But having that conversation before the end arrives is hard. And this is why, as intensive care professionals, we sometimes need to lead the way and ask people for their views on these topics in a non-confrontational, open manner. A heartbreaking, difficult two-week stay in intensive care, treating futility, is no substitute for an honest conversation with a patient who has the right to express their wishes about their life and death. Perhaps if we spoke more about our own deaths, it might make the end of our lives a little bit better.

And so, for Seren, if the heart of a frail, elderly nursing home resident stopped beating, this was not because of a new problem that could easily be fixed. It was part of a natural chain of predictable events. The cause of death would be a long life. In these cases, CPR would not prolong life, only extend death. She was brilliant at her job; the residents loved her.

Yet with Kai it was completely different. Kai was not

that frail, wise old man in Dylan Thomas's poem. He was a young man and in great health. Until he died. There had been a new problem, something that could be fixed. So CPR was exactly the right thing to do.

After arriving at hospital by ambulance, doctors carried out hundreds of tests to find out what had happened to Kai. The blood supply to his heart was fine – no heart attack. The electrical circuits that carry impulses were working normally too. There were no blood clots in his lungs, no bleeds on his brain. Instead, the cause of Kai's death was also life – a busy life. Trying to do everything, for everyone, all of the time. He had travelled to the Old Flour Mill cottage after a busy night shift, drank coffee to get him through the day, not eaten much, not drunk much, played with the kids, carried the cases, caught up with his friends. Even in the weeks before, Kai had juggled endless projects at work, visited his parents, done renovation projects at home. In the months before, there had been Covid, work, more work, and a busy family life. Like many doctors, especially intensive care doctors, Kai was also a perfectionist. Not for himself, but for others. He didn't want to let people down, took on more than his arms could carry, and when he dropped something, he would figure out a way to pick it back up, balancing it on top of the pile.

After all that, no wonder Kai ended up falling off.

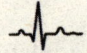

Good advice can come from unexpected places. When the retired former world number one tennis player Roger Federer stepped on to the stage at Dartmouth college in New Hampshire, the audience of recent graduates from the Ivy League establishment didn't know what to expect. Yet despite it being only the second time Federer had ever been on a college campus after leaving school at sixteen, he gave world number one advice. His message was just what Kai needed to hear.

Federer looked perfect on the sunny, green New Hampshire day – luminous white collar around his neck on top of a velvet black robe. Every hair in place, with shiny skin, white teeth and a wide smile. But Federer's message was the opposite – there is no such thing as perfection. Perfection does not exist.

Drawing on data and not just feelings, Federer explained how, although he won 80 per cent of matches during his 28-year professional career, he actually lost 46 per cent of all points. And more importantly, after losing these points, he just had to move on. Not dwell. If professional tennis players ruminated on every point that they lose, they would lose the whole game and then the match. A point is just a point. When faced with challenges in life, do confront them with your whole best. But when that point is over, it is over. Move on. And give your best to the next, and then the next after that.

'When you're playing a point, it is the most important thing in the world,' he explained. 'But the truth is, whatever game you play in life, sometimes you're going to lose. A point, a match, a season, a job: it's a roller coaster, with many ups and downs.'

The speech was covered by the world's media, but they failed to recognise the thick, textured brown tree stump that Federer was standing behind. This was a memorial to the 'Lone Pine' tree, a gathering place for graduates in Dartmouth since 1829 until the original tree was struck by lightning in 1895. The stump on which Federer placed his hands allows us to remember what was there before. The stump is strong and stable, yet it has no roots. The original couldn't be fixed after the lightning strike. So it is now far from perfect. But it was perfect to speak behind. It is instead held in place by its own weight pressing on the ground below. Like trees, humans are gardens to tend, not machines to fix.

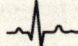

And so the cause of Kai's death was eventually put down to not one thing but many. Life is rarely as simple as A goes to B. His lack of sleep, working hard, being dehydrated, some wine, lots of coffee, eating late and Kai's already slow resting heart rate led to what could have been his end. Instead, it was a new beginning. Sometimes, you are not stressed only because you are doing too much; you are stressed because you are doing too little of what makes you feel alive.

Kai couldn't drive for six months, something that had a profound impact on his life and family. Everyday tasks like shopping, school drop-offs and commuting to work became major challenges, requiring him to rely on the kindness of colleagues and friends. The overwhelming support from family, friends and even strangers left Kai and his wife deeply moved. The nurses at work even pooled money to gift his family a weekend getaway, highlighting just how much this experience impacted them all, both in struggles and in the kindness they received.

Kai originally told me I should be speaking with Seren not him. He almost felt like an imposter in his own death. He felt his story shouldn't feature because he was not that different. But during our conversation I think a realisation came over him: 'My family do say I'm different.'

Kai 2.0 is no longer travelling at 120mph. Although he is still at 100mph, that is still a big difference. He balances fewer things on the pile held in his arms. When things drop, he often leaves them on the floor. In the three months it took Kai to get back to work, he lent on others around him more. Friends sent food and best wishes; he made some time for himself without feeling guilty. As a family they made some big decisions. They packed up a city life and moved to the coast even though their new home was over two hours from Kai's work. They went anyway; they made it work. And when Kai did return to his ICU, he quit some roles to make room for another.

Kai now organises gatherings of healthcare professionals – from senior consultants to junior nurses – to learn from patients who have died or had a difficult healthcare journey.

We call these 'Morbidity and mortality' (M&M) meetings, where each case is presented as a story with people bringing their own insights and experiences. Beyond practical learning, M&M meetings provide a space for emotional processing, fostering a culture of continuous improvement and transparency. That is why Kai started calling them M&M&M – morbidity, mortality and merit – the final 'M' recognising what was done well, be it saving a life or helping the family of a dying relative. Even when immediate improvements are not evident, sharing and reflecting can be therapeutic. It helps professionals process the emotional weight of their work, acknowledge their humanity, and find solace in shared experiences. M&M meetings thus enhance patient safety and nurture the resilience and growth of caregivers, blending practical improvement with emotional support. Subconscious or not, Kai is now leading something that he has gone through, to help others.

And the lessons that come from M&M meetings are often not about doing more and more. They are often about doing less and less, but better. I like to say to students struggling with what to do next with a complex patient, 'Don't just do something, stand there!' Just as Kai made significant changes in his life, Eddie Cantor, a Broadway performer, humanitarian and founder of the March of Dimes, an organisation that helped defeat polio through vaccination, once said, 'Slow down and enjoy life. It's not only the scenery you miss by going too fast – you also miss the sense of where you are going and why.' This is not about having less or doing less. It's about making room for more of what matters. Quitting is the best way of succeeding. Or as Federer has shown us, winners are just people who know how to lose better.

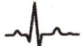

Sundays used to be a drag in our house. They would start with an argument with my daughter to practise the piano, starting with mild threats of technology removal and ending with bribes. After a few minutes of hearing major notes that should have been minor, she would inevitably ask, 'Can I quit?' Given the time and money already invested in her lessons and books, my response was always a firm, 'No!' I believed she just needed more persistence. More grit.

On Monday morning at work, like Kai I'd channel this persistence. I would keep doing the projects I've been postponing, act in roles I'd outgrown. Some of us do entire jobs that merely fill time. We don't quit. We endure. Because quitting carries a stigma. We focus on the time already invested, the progress made, and the commitments we've made.

One Sunday, I cracked. 'Fine, quit then!' I said to my daughter, throwing the piano books to the ground. I expected her to relent, but she didn't. She knew better than me. She instead redirected her time to something she genuinely enjoyed and excelled at – dancing. Now, Sundays are filled with joy. She loves dancing, she's good at it, and it makes her feel more like herself. The girl who took over her spot at the oversubscribed piano class is happier too. Sometimes the solution is not persistence but knowing when to quit.

As leaders, we're often taught that quitting equals failure. Yet, true leadership involves helping others thrive. Good leaders should know when to lead and, more importantly, when to shut up and listen. Those we lead need opportunities to grow, spaces to fill. What if you are occupying one of those spaces? In Tim Harford's podcast *Cautionary Tales*, he explores how Nobel Prize winners, known for their perseverance, often have a wider array of superficial interests than their peers. They move in and out of different pursuits, quitting more frequently.

Persistence has its place, of course. It's vital at times. The key is to use it wisely. Focus on what you love, what you're good at, or what makes you feel more like you. Dance if you're a dancer, not a pianist. Simultaneously, let go of projects you know you'll never finish. Quit roles that have grown stale, allowing others to take them on with fresh energy. Consider the opportunities missed by clinging to things you don't truly want, rather than the time already spent on them. Embrace the joy of missing out (JOMO), let go of the fear of missing out (FOMO). I also advocate for the joy of walking out (JOWO). Embrace quitting. You're never too old to learn the piano, but you're also never too old to find joy in walking away from what no longer serves you. Less grit, more quit.

Despite the changes in Kai's life, the biggest adjustment since that day in the Old Flour Mill cottage wasn't for him, it was for others. But this too is an essential lesson – realise what a massive impact you have on others. Living our life is not just about living our life. Others live through you, and your words and your deeds change other lives as much, if not more than your own.

Realising the impact the events had had on their family and friends, when Kai's family next went away, they spotted an old phone box transformed into a place to house a defibrillator by Community HeartBeat Trust, a charity dedicated to increasing the number of public access defibrillators in rural parts of the UK. These famous red 'Jubilee kiosk' phone boxes were launched in 1936 to celebrate King George V's Silver Jubilee. By the '60s almost 70,000 kiosks could be found across the countryside. The charity is changing these into life-saving devices.

The transformation of phone boxes to house defibrillators is a powerful metaphor for how we can change and improve our own lives. Just as technology evolves to meet new needs, we too can repurpose our skills, habits and perspectives to create a more fulfilling and impactful existence. Embracing change rather than resisting it allows us to discover new opportunities. Recognise and leverage your unique strengths and experiences, even those that seem outdated or irrelevant. These can be the foundation for new, innovative paths that give your life meaning and direction, especially when they impact on the lives of others. But to do this we all need to regularly think about our skills, habits and experiences. Death is the ultimate way to do this, but you don't have to die. In fact, it is best not to.

The selfie that Kai's growing family of five took outside that transformed phone box was sent to everyone who had been on that memorable reunion trip. By the time the family arrived home a few days later, there was a single postcard on the doormat. It was addressed to 'Dr D Fib', with the selfie as the main photo with large capital letters spelling the word 'CLEAR' on the other side. It had been sent by the surgeon who had laughed at Kai's joke, 'If I did die, I can tell you now that there's nothing back there!'

Kai had been wrong, there is something after death – the people you leave behind whose roots you have helped nurture. Life after death is all about living on in the memories of those who knew you. So, live a life worth remembering and make sure to leave behind stories that are too good to forget.

9

Heartless

Rhys, forty-two years old
Cause of death: Rugby
Cause of life: Self-forgiveness

The first time I saw Rhys Thomas, he was wearing a blood-red Welsh rugby jersey, playing against Italy at the 75,000-capacity Millennium Stadium in Cardiff. It was his fourth of an eventual seven caps playing for Wales. The second time I met Rhys was at a cafe near his home, only this time he didn't have a heartbeat.

Born in Johannesburg to his Welsh engineer dad and artist mum, childhood was spent outdoors, climbing trees and playing cricket with his large band of cousins. His early flair for sport took Rhys to the premier government-run King Edward VII School in the Houghton Estate in Johannesburg. The long list of professional sports stars and business leaders it has produced is a testament to the values, discipline and structure it gave to boarders like Rhys. And he needed these boundaries – his wild streak could then be focused on sport rather than crime or drugs.

'It was like the military just without the killing,' he told me.

But the school did have plenty of violence. 'It broke a lot of people, the lashings and the beatings, never from the teachers but from the older boys. And then a few years later you were those older boys, you were giving out the punishments.' The school made Rhys into the man he would become, but later it would lead to his downfall.

As a cricket-mad 13-year-old, Rhys watched South Africa's victory in the 1995 Rugby World Cup on a big television with his cousins. The country, still reeling from the apartheid era, was in desperate need of a unifying moment and so was he. The weight of history and the hope of a nation were on the shoulders of the Springboks. When Nelson Mandela stepped on to the field wearing the green and gold jersey, the roar of the crowd was deafening, a sound that seemed to echo the breaking of old barriers.

As the final whistle blew, confirming South Africa's triumph over New Zealand, Rhys's family home erupted in jubilation. It wasn't just a sports victory; it was a symbolic win for unity and reconciliation. People of all races were hugging, crying and celebrating together. But for Rhys, the meaning was different. It made him pick up a rugby ball for the first time, leaving his cricket bat behind as he returned to school after the holidays. Within ten years of

Rhys scoring his first try against his school's arch rival, the nearby St John's private school, Rhys was wearing that red Welsh jersey in front of a roaring crowd.

The decision to move across the world for sport was a tough one. In the weeks before he signed a rugby contract, Rhys was offered the chance to live on a kibbutz in Gaza. But seeing a Welsh rugby team on tour in Johannesburg playing strip touch rugby, laughing and running around naked as the sun set on the beach, helped seal the decision for fun-loving Rhys. He was soon stepping off a plane wearing shorts and flip-flops into the wet Welsh winter.

Rhys had signed a contract to play rugby for the large, industrial Welsh town of Newport. It was quite a culture shock. He thought there had been a mix-up when he was dropped off at the waterlogged training pitch, covered in a strange substance he had never seen before – mud. Although Newport has a rich history and strong sense of community, the city's struggles extend beyond just the weather. Newport has several areas that rank among the most underprivileged in Wales and in the top 10 per cent most deprived areas in the UK. The average life expectancy is three years lower than in rural Monmouthshire just 10 miles away. Newport is still the only place I have ever been where I have seen a dog step on a human shit.

Despite the dramatic acclimatisation, Rhys was soon called up for the Wales Under-21 side, helping them win the Six Nations in his final season. He was selected for the World Cup Dream Team as the best tight-head prop, before putting on the Welsh jersey as a professional for the first time against Argentina in June 2006.

'There is nothing in the world like playing rugby in Wales. My heart pounded as I pulled that red jersey over my head and felt the Welsh crest against my chest for the first time. There were 75,000 people singing the national anthem, flames shooting over the green grass as I emerged on to the pitch into a war of sport for eighty amazing minutes.'

But like so many at the top of their game, with the biggest highs come the lowest lows. Rhys had been injected into Wales as an 18-year-old, rising to superstardom. After the games came the parties, the free drinks, the temptations around every corner. The disciplined walls of his school crumbled, the physical abuse replaced by a brutal training regime, but his wild streak was no longer satisfied by his pitch-time alone. During untamed nights out, Rhys would do things he would regret and say things he didn't mean. If drinking alcohol is like borrowing happiness from tomorrow, Rhys became overcome by debt – he owed much to his team, his family and himself. He would carry this past behaviour on a long, difficult journey with him until he finally learned to become a better, stronger man. But he would need to be broken first.

The cracks started after a punishing blow to his chest during a very physical game. This sparked a series of events that led to Rhys's heart stopping twice before he was able to scrape his life back together. But the life Rhys returned to would be unrecognisably good in some way, but unrecognisably bad in others.

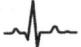

It is not just professional sports stars who have their demons – doctors like me rarely live the life they advise. The media had a party when England's new health secretary, Thérèse Coffey, was photographed smoking a cigar while clutching a flute of champagne. But I'm also certainly not 100 per cent healthy nor 100 per cent moral – on a good day I may hit 50 per cent. Healthcare workers tend to drink to hazardous levels more frequently than the general population, with over 20 per cent also being smokers. I remember feeling guilty caring for a critically injured cyclist after riding to work that morning not wearing a helmet. I've spoken to a family about alcoholism while sucking a mint to disguise last night's afterparty. But is it okay for a heart surgeon to smoke or the hepatologist to drink whisky? More generally, as life becomes overexposed, spilling all of our inner personal lives on the floor of the town square through social media, how should we deal with our own hypocrisy?

David Fleming, a cultural historian and economist, stated in his book *Lean Logic*, 'There is no reason why he should not argue for standards better than he manages to achieve in his own life.' I am no paragon of perfect living but can still be a coach guiding patients to do better than I. José Mourinho played fewer than 100 games in Portugal's second division. Arrigo Sacchi, despite being one of the greatest ever football managers, never played professionally.

Of course, there may be boundaries to avoid, but we are all complex and multifaceted. To echo Bob Dylan, who was channelling Walt Whitman, we are full of contradictions and many moods. We all contain multitudes. And that is okay. Or perhaps it is even better than perfection, advising on perfection. Carl Sagan, one of the most celebrated scientists of the past 100 years, famously said, 'We are made of star-stuff.' That sounds inspiring and it is. We are all recycled from something else, it just depends on how far you want to go back. The iron in our blood was formed inside a giant red star billions of years ago. But since then, it has moved through countless rocks, mountains, trees and butterflies. How beautiful. But your iron has also moved through guns, bullets that have killed, bacteria that have infected others, and steel that has spilt blood. As Fleming aptly concludes in his book, 'Indeed, it would be worrying if his ideals were not better than the way he lives.'

After the severe impact to his chest, Rhys needed weeks of painkillers and steroid injections to ease the pain. But even when the bruising settled, things weren't right. Rhys would get pain in his jaw, causing him to grind his teeth at night. During training, his left arm would feel tight and his heart would pound like when he first wore that red Welsh jersey, especially after drinking high-dose caffeine shots that were a standard part of the training regime.

This culminated in a heart attack after a game, needing

Rhys to take six months off rugby entirely. But he was then given the all-clear to return to professional sport and by 2012, life was finally looking up. His rugby was the strongest it had been for years, his fitness was back, and his mind was sharp. He was about to sign the contract of a lifetime with French team Biarritz, known for its rich history and strong rugby traditions.

Although life can kick you when you are down, being on top of the world means there is further to fall. Five years after his heart attack, Rhys felt great, at the top of his game. The day before his mum's birthday, recovery from a minor neck injury meant Rhys needed to be at the gym earlier than the rest of the team. His 'easy' warm-up of 1,000 calories on the bike in forty-five minutes was coming to an end. At minute forty-three, the final few calories ticked by when the familiar feelings of neck, jaw and arm pain returned. Rhys's vision faded as he stumbled off the bike into the team physiotherapist's office. Crumbling on to the floor, an ambulance was called as Rhys lay still, sweating, his face moist like the grease inside a pizza box, having a massive heart attack.

At the hospital, doctors tried to open up the blood vessels around his heart using wires threaded through the artery in his right wrist. As they did, the blood supply to his heart muscle reduced even further and his heart started to fail. Doctors rushed Rhys to the cardiac theatre, stopping his heart on purpose to perform an emergency quadruple bypass. As Rhys's chest was opened by the surgeons, they saw the main blood vessel to his heart had split open, caused by the blow to his chest years before, combined with the physical stress of training, caffeine and his lifestyle. Rhys's heart muscle was severely thinned at the front and could no longer beat. The last words that the muscular, powerful, 'wild' sportsman Rhys said to his family, including his children aged between four and eighteen, before having surgery were simple – 'I love you.'

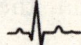

The phrase 'all you need is love' often gets dismissed as a clichéd sentiment. But allowing it to extend beyond the boundaries of a 'boy meets girl' romantic love story makes it hit home. Although articles espouse the rise of toxic masculinity, the truth is that even Rhys – a solid, South African rugby player brought up on corporal punishment at school – chose love as his final message before facing his end.

Perhaps the Beatles were pointing towards research showing that married couples do indeed tend to live longer than their single counterparts. This is largely attributed to the social and emotional support inherent in a long-term union. A partner can provide accountability for healthy lifestyle behaviours, resulting in lower rates of substance abuse, lower blood pressure and reduced levels of depression compared to single peers. However, recent studies have shown that these longevity benefits are not exclusive to romantic relationships. Similar advantages can be found in close, non-romantic relationships that offer a degree of emotional support and 'love'. These findings suggest that the quality of social connections, rather than the specific nature of the relationship, is crucial for fostering long-term health and well-being.

Up until 2013, no human deaths had occurred due to wind turbine accidents. That changed on 29 October 2013, when two of the four mechanics servicing a wind turbine in Ooltgensplaat, Netherlands, were killed. A fire broke out at the top of the turbine after a short circuit. Due to the height of the turbine and location of the fire, the fire department had trouble extinguishing the blaze. A specialised team were called in to use a large crane to battle the raging fire. Two of the mechanics were able to escape but the remaining two, men aged nineteen and twenty-one, became trapped on the top of the turbine. In their final moments they didn't jump or scream. Instead, an iconic image of Daan Kous and Arjan Kortus showed them hugging before the black smoke and flames engulfed their bodies. Love isn't all you need, but it is all we think about when there is little else left.

Rhys's heart remained silent and still for hours as surgeons replaced the blood vessels on its surface during a difficult operation. Blood to his other organs flowed through a large heart-lung machine as the team realised that over half of his heart's muscle had died after his previous chest injury and the heart attack that followed. His blood pressure was too low to come off the bypass machine and so surgeons needed to insert a balloon into Rhys's aorta to keep enough blood flowing.

A SECOND ACT

When Rhys woke in the Intensive Care Unit, with his body fighting to stay alive, his brain starved of oxygen, the dreams he experienced were indistinguishable from reality. The ceiling of the ward turned into waves of hot sand, his wife appeared as a figurehead at the front of a pirate ship. Rhys experienced past and possible future lives, while trapped in a cyclical reality that felt like it lasted decades. But even when he was discharged from hospital two weeks later, life would not get much easier.

In a heartbeat, Rhys had been transformed from an elite, professional sportsman into a frail, dependent shell who couldn't even walk to the toilet. His heart struggled to squeeze; he suffered crippling panic attacks that could only be calmed by breathing techniques he was taught at hospital. But when even this breath work stopped working, the only treatment was one of the world's most popular, destructive drugs – alcohol. Rhys fell into his self-destructive former ways and rather than alcohol helping him get through the day, it started to make his condition even worse. His heart function was declining day by day and within months, Rhys was on the urgent heart transplant waiting list. He was given twelve months to live, but as the months ticked down, no heart could be found. Instead, after nine months of waiting Rhys was given a stark choice – become a man without a heartbeat and live or keep your own heartbeat and die.

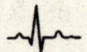

Nearly every mammal, large and small, shares a fascinating relationship between its average life expectancy and its heartbeat. This link gifts mammals roughly 1 billion heartbeats in their lifetime. For instance, a hummingbird's heart, which races at more than 1,200 beats per minute, gives it a lifespan of merely three to five years. Conversely, the blue whale's heart, which beats only about six times per minute, supports a life expectancy of more than 100 years. Humans, however, have artificially extended their lifespan through medical advancements, averaging around 3 billion heartbeats over a lifetime.

When you dash to catch a bus or do a workout at the gym your heart rate surges. Even if you are not a fitness fanatic, in a typical six-minute period of sex, your normal 400 beats will rise to more than 1,000. Not only does your heart beat faster, but it also contracts more forcefully, expelling 120 millilitres of blood per beat compared to the usual 80 millilitres. This change boosts the blood volume pumped through your body from 30 litres to more than 120 litres. But when your heart fails like Rhys's, it can't adapt to changes. Rhys's heart struggled to just beat at a normal pace, ejecting only half of the normal amounts of blood. So, activities as minor as walking to the toilet would starve Rhys's muscles of oxygen.

Medicine has long been captivated by the heart, ever since William Harvey described it as 'the circuit of the blood' in 1649. What is essentially a pump is both soft and responsive, yet robust and enduring. Yet, like all pumps, it can fail. Medicine soon came up with options for repair.

The methods designed to repair blood vessels that were used during Rhys's bypass operation were developed by the Lebanese-American surgeon Dr Michael DeBakey. His life was nothing short of special. He discovered early links between smoking and lung cancer, performed one of the world's first heart-bypass surgeries and introduced operations still essential to save lives in my hospital today. He even trialled the first mechanical heart device that is now fast becoming a reasonable alternative to a heart transplant for some patients like Rhys. DeBakey continued working until the age of ninety-nine after suffering a catastrophic aneurysm rupture himself aged ninety-seven. His life was saved by a seven-hour operation that he had invented, followed by a prolonged stay in the ICU. He died two months before his one hundredth birthday.

For some patients, simply replacing the pipes that supply blood to the heart is not enough. When heart muscle dies it does not regenerate. While heart transplants offer a lifeline, they are fraught with challenges. Finding a suitable donor match in time can be difficult, and post-transplant life involves a commitment to powerful immunosuppressive drugs that prevent rejection but can cause severe infections and even cancer.

Three hundred years after Harvey described the heart's wonder, advances in medical technology have produced mechanical devices to help the failing heart that are small enough to be implanted under the skin. The evolution of heart support devices has been groundbreaking. The first heart-bypass operation on a human, in 1951, was unsuccessful, but by 1953, the iron heart machine saved an 18-year-old woman at Thomas Jefferson University Hospital in Philadelphia by closing a hole in her heart. But now, these devices can sustain life for extended periods even in those with minimal heart function. These machines have even been inserted during a cardiac arrest in the Louvre, Paris. The *Mona Lisa* silently looked on as French medical teams put the patient on a heart-lung bypass machine in the middle of the museum.

Remarkably, it is now possible to live without a heart entirely. Former Czech firefighter Jakub Halik was the first, living for six months with two mechanical pumps instead of a heart, and even managing to visit the gym despite having no pulse. This was the choice that doctors gave Rhys. A transplant could not be found for him in time so he could opt to live with a mechanical pump or not live at all.

In the UK, the shortage of hearts and other organs for transplant is a critical issue, leaving many patients in desperate need. With more than 300 people waiting for a heart transplant, the demand far surpasses the supply. Despite the 2020 implementation of the opt-out donation system across the UK, the gap remains wide, particularly affecting those with urgent needs. The wait can be excruciatingly long, with many patients on mechanical heart support struggling to maintain their quality of life. It is even longer in minority ethnic groups where consent rates for donation are particularly low despite the increased need in those communities. This is due to a combination of factors. Genetic diversity between people means that finding a specific tissue type, the protein fingerprints in our organs, is harder in minority groups under-represented as donors. Hence there are fewer compatible organs. Additionally, historical mistrust of healthcare systems and some cultural beliefs can lower registration as organ donors in some communities. Socioeconomic challenges, such as limited access to healthcare, also contribute to lower donation rates.

This was why I acted as an ambassador for the 'Tribute to Life' project, launched by the NHS Blood and Transplant service, at the 2022 Commonwealth Games in Birmingham. This aims to enhance ethical organ donation and transplantation practices across nations. By fostering international co-operation, the project seeks to improve organ donation rates and save lives through shared learning and collaboration. It was at the planning session at the House of Lords that I sat next to one of the heart surgeons who implanted Rhys's artificial heart.

But it doesn't have to be this way. Think about your closest loved one right now – maybe your son or daughter, your mum or your dad. Imagine the feeling when the phone rings offering them another chance at life through the gift of donation. Imagine that same phone call saying that the gift has instead been cremated or buried in a box. Donation is not only the greatest gift that can be given, but it is a gift that is of no value unless it is given. Intensive care facilitates this most selfless human act. We care for the physical body of a patient, even after their soul has departed when their brainstem, the part that makes you legally alive, has died. We protect their organs, ensuring their donation has the maximum benefit to recipients who may live hundreds of miles away. Although these people will never have met the donor, their second shot at life can be a constant reminder to us all of how far humanity and medicine have come.

I hope that Chapter 8 can save a life through teaching you CPR. But I hope this chapter can save even more lives if just one of you considers what to leave behind after your death. Think about how what you no longer need could transform the lives of many others. Once you have thought about this, no matter the outcome, tell your family about your wishes. Death need not detract from the joy of living. Even in death you can leave a legacy of hope for others.

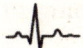

The team explained to Rhys how a mechanical device could be fitted inside his failing heart, attached to a battery pack worn over his shoulder, to give an extra boost to every heartbeat. Although this would improve the health of his organs, Rhys would lose all pulses in his body as the pump would smooth out the blood flow into a continuous stream. With just months left to live, Rhys had little choice. He spent a traumatic six weeks waiting in the cardiac ward, watching many older and younger patients die before or after similar procedures. He became familiar with the ebb and flow of life and of death. First, an emergency buzzer would sound in the bed next to him. Soon, the medical team would rush in and try various treatments. Sometimes they worked, often they did not. When they did not, the patient would die. Curtains were pulled around, families cried, the body moved, the bed wiped clean, curtains opened, ready to receive another patient. Rhys waited his turn to go on the conveyer belt of life.

But the day of his operation did come. He kissed his family goodbye, told them he loved them once again, and was taken to theatre. This time the operation did not go according to plan. The scar tissue from his previous surgery meant it took three heart surgeons over four hours just to get near his heart. But after nearly twelve hours on the bypass machine, a member of the theatre team came to tell Rhys's family that they hadn't been able to put the device in his heart. They were going to wake Rhys up and move to end-of-life care. A knock on the family room door mid-conversation interrupted them with news of a breakthrough. They had just managed to divide the delicate, thin muscle remaining in his heart and slip the metal limbs of the device into position.

After two weeks in intensive care, Rhys needed a tracheostomy, meaning he was unable to speak when his eyes finally opened. Instead, a nurse gave him a clipboard to write on. That clipboard still hangs in Rhys's house today, reminding him what is important and what was at stake. Scrawled in thick black pen are the words 'I love you'.

We forget how machines, drugs and procedures can fix many parts of a person, but not the whole. I can sometimes save a life, but not fix a life. In the weeks that followed Rhys's operation, he spiralled to new lows. His purpose in life, his job, his security, his identity had all be taken away. He was living on benefits and the six weeks spent in the cardiac ward watching the supermarket of life and death would return in the early hours of the morning, invading Rhys's thoughts. He couldn't sleep, he couldn't think straight. He only found one effective treatment – alcohol.

Rhys started drinking to blackout levels again. All of the things he had held dear were collateral damage as his relationships broke down. Then he was taken off the transplant list. His behaviour was so self-destructive that he would wake up in police cells to the noise of his new mechanical heart beeping. Its batteries would last only eight hours before Rhys had just fifteen minutes to change or charge the unit once the alarm sounded. If it ran out, Rhys would die.

'I was angry and bitter. I was a victim, and I didn't care about anything. I didn't have the energy even for my emotions. And when I got that low, I could see no way out. I had done so much wrong; how could I ever do good?'

The rock bottom would come in 2019 when a car accident after drinking led to Rhys being taken to a rehab facility in South Africa by his family. We have all had that feeling of being in a stationary car, stopped at green lights. You need someone to honk their horn at you from behind. For Rhys, this was his last chance at his dog-eared life. But can people really change? Should we carry around our old mistakes like baggage, letting them weigh us down as punishment? The question Rhys asked more than any other during his month in rehab was, 'Who am I?'

I have spoken with many people who have made poor 'choices' in life. These choices often end in ICU. The more I listen to their stories, the more I question the role free will has in people's predicaments. Although my mum and dad are very proud of my achievements, are these really of just my making? I didn't choose to be born into a loving family, into a household full of books, in a country with free education or in a century when most babies survive. I didn't mix my personal blend of neurotransmitters in my brain that means I can understand science, avoid addiction and turn away from violence. And any choices I make occur against a backdrop of overwhelming noise and chaos in the world around me, making it feel as though personal decisions are insignificant in the grand scheme of things. Even MRI studies now show that our subconscious processes predetermine so-called choices long before we are consciously aware of making them. If there were any doubt before, this reinforces why medical care should never be allocated based only on the perceived worth of a person. Even if your life is a series of great decisions, should you be judged only by your worst one? If so, who really are you? It seems simple, but does anyone really know who they are?

The Oxford philosopher Derek Parfit spent more than twenty-five years trying to answer this question. The explanation he settled on could help Rhys and millions like him who struggle to walk away from the shadows of their past.

Parfit argued that personal identity is not what really matters when thinking about who we are. Instead, psychological continuity and connectedness are crucial. 'You' are not a static entity but a series of interconnected experiences that change and warp with time. We are not even the same person throughout our lives, instead we live life as a series of evolving selves. And while this highbrow notion seems of little relevance to a hard-hitting rugby player with an addiction like Rhys, it can be life-saving. You can let go of the past. You can be someone else. You are someone else. Every day. You can forgive yourself and become anew. Your past self does not define your future.

But shouldn't identity matter? Yes, I am very different from my 18-year-old spotty, thinner self but still feel responsible for the stupid things I did back then because I am the same person. And I also care about what may happen to me when I am sixty because that's also going to be me. Parfit agrees that yes, you should care about your past and future selves, but not because you are literally the same person. I will have the same name, the same birthmark on my ankle. I've been walking around in the same flesh-bag body since being born and have many of the same likes and dislikes.

But, Parfit argues, it is not these physical things that matter. Instead, his ideas align with the ancient philosophical puzzle known as the Ship of Theseus. Imagine gradually replacing every part of a ship day-by-day. You change all of the wooden planks, swap out every nut and bolt, until one day, decades later, none of the original components remain. Is it still the same ship? In fact, every seven years, each cell in your body has already been replaced. Are you then the same person? Parfit uses this analogy to illustrate his view that identity is not tied to a specific set of components but rather to the continuity and connection between them over time. It also shows how we should consider our actions against what Parfit calls 'future persons', the generations that come after us.

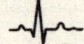

Healthcare is responsible for around 5 per cent of all greenhouse gas emissions. If it were a country, medicine would be the fifth-highest polluter, ironic given the impact that climate change has on the burdens of ill health. It's hard to raise a glass to the next decade while the climate emergency causes more deaths than smoking, AIDS, diabetes and vehicle crashes combined. These climate-related illnesses and injuries disproportionately affect low-income communities – another example of the poorest and most vulnerable people bearing the largest burden of ill health.

And within that polluting country, ICU would be the industrial heartland of emissions, a carbon hotspot in the hospital, producing three times more output compared with general wards. Every cardiac arrest patient in this book needs the equivalent electricity of a four-person household per day with over 180kg^2 of CO_2 produced, the same as burning 80 litres of petrol. The machines used to care for a critically ill patient require three times as much energy per day as the average family home uses per day. We would need to plant over 70,000 trees to absorb our unit's carbon footprint and wait 80 years for them to reach their maximum carbon uptake. But that is OK. Or put another way, as the Greek proverb tells us, "A society grows great when old people plant trees whose shade they shall never sit in."

Alarm is all very well, but what about solutions? I spend a lot of my time at overseas medical conferences and as I fly home it's embarrassing that my talk about respiratory disease was powered by jet fuel, while the calories provided by the conference were delivered through meat. The lights that brought my colourful slides of battered lungs to life took their energy from the coal that coated the insides of the patient I was trying to save.

I want organisers of these events to commit to providing food that doesn't bloat the atmosphere as well as those eating it. A meat-free lunch would do little to dampen spirits but could hopefully be a start to dampening forest fires over the next decade. A quarter of global emissions come from food production — half of them from animal product emissions, chiefly beef and lamb. Livestock contributes to global warming not only through methane production but through deforestation linked to expanded pastures, and the Intergovernmental Panel on Climate Change is pleading for us to switch to a plant-based diet.

If air travel is unavoidable in allowing human connections at conferences, we should nudge speakers to use honorariums or travel costs to cover ethical carbon offsetting projects, and this should be built into the travel expenses policy.

Organisers could cover travel costs of only the most efficient airlines or advocate train travel for short-haul alternatives. With online streaming and virtual connections, travelling halfway around the world to watch someone present slides and to check your emails at the back of a lecture theatre seems a little odd.

And the venues should be chosen not only for delegates' convenience but also to improve our lives now and those of future generations. Selecting facilities that commit to renewable energy is a price worth paying for organisers, delegates and the planet.

This is also slowly being tackled for patients in ICU. Simply reducing unnecessary blood tests across Australia has saved $33 million, 4,400 litres of blood and the labour equal to forty full-time staff, not to mention the environmental benefits. My own unit now turns computers off overnight, uses light-emitting diode bulbs, and has stopped fully charging unnecessary electrical equipment. We used to spend more than £100,000 per year on those terrible plastic non-sterile gloves, 100 pairs used every day on every patient – 4,000 pairs a day in total. Reducing inappropriate gloves use by 20 per cent, bringing back human touch and good handwashing instead, has saved more than £20,000 and the burden of 1.5 million pairs of plastic waste from these gloves every year.

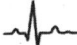

Nelson Mandela, like the Ship of Theseus, changed the cells in his body as he aged, changed his views, his knowledge and his relationships as he journeyed from prisoner to president. When he held up that rugby trophy watched by 13-year-old Rhys, he was a testament to profound change. 'Do not judge me by my successes, judge me by how many times I fell down and got back up again,' he would later say.

In other words, personal identity is not what matters. What matters is psychological continuity and connectedness. And as we age, we have fewer and fewer psychological connections with our childhood selves. Our distant future selves also become less connected to our present selves. I might even be more connected to other people, my wife and my children, than I am to that 18-year-old Matt Morgan.

This is a powerful realisation. It gives us permission and a logical argument to allow us to move on. You will still drag your flesh-bag body with the scars from your past mistakes but realise now that you are more like the person that you have become than any loser from the past. Or as C. S. Lewis said, 'You can't go back and change the beginning, but you can start where you are and change the ending.'

Although Rhys is not an Oxford philosopher, he is living proof of Parfit's conclusion. His stay in rehab gave him the tools, the time and the humanity to heal. When we met on a sunny Welsh morning in a cafe in his hometown of Caerleon, I was the only one drinking anything. As I sipped a strong coffee, still tired from a colleague's retirement party that weekend, Rhys was a picture of health. Physically he was the lightest he had ever been, sober for five years and not even drinking coffee. As I shook his hand, I couldn't resist feeling for his pulse in the wrist still scarred from his procedures. Still nothing. It was an unnerving experience, talking and laughing with someone despite them having no heartbeat. But around his shoulder was the telltale black strap holding his lifeline device making this possible.

Although Rhys was back on the transplant list, he was in a difficult place – too well to be in the super-urgent category, but too unwell to live much longer without a transplant. He is approaching the world record of living with an artificial heart for fourteen years.

'I'm still training as hard as ever, every day. But this is for the game of my life. I need to stay my best to make it to the starting fifteen to get my transplant. I want to keep living.'

He fitted perfectly into his new skin. He hasn't forgotten about the past; he owns it and can still look back at that wild Rhys. But he can also gaze forwards, letting his life move on to better things. His website is framed by a widescreen colour photo of a strong, confident man, barefoot and tattooed, standing on top of a Welsh mountain, looking out across the scattered clouds with the sun just breaking through.

The breath work that got him through his panic attacks in hospital has led to a new passion teaching leaders in business and sport this life skill to address their own demons. His work with the charity Sporting Chance, founded by the former England football captain Tony Adams, allowed Rhys to share his journey with other professional athletes, supporting their own emotional and health problems. This lit a flame inside Rhys to set up his own charity, Tidy Butt, that deals with the stigma around mental health in schools, businesses and professional sports teams across Wales.

After we had spent a few hours together, I asked Rhys the last question on my list: 'If you could press a button right now that would stop you from ever having become ill, would you press it?'

'No way,' came Rhys's answer, without missing a beat. 'I miss rugby so much and I would love to play again. Perhaps I will after my transplant,' he smiled. 'But I have found my sobriety. I found who I really am. Who I can be.

'The best record I've broken is not a sporting one. I've broken multigenerational links of addiction in my family.

I've changed the space between now and the future for me and my family.'

We can all learn from that space. First, we need to find space. There is a big difference between being mindful and having your mind full. Victor Frankl's spectacular book, *Man's Search for Meaning*, that inspired Jack to plant trees in Chapter 2 includes the line 'Between stimulus and response there is a space. In that space is our power to choose our response. In our response lies our growth and our freedom.'

He also went on to say, 'When no longer able to change a situation, we are challenged to change ourselves.'

Rhys is now a strong, fit, happy and confident leader. He is one of the most successful people to have ever come from that school in South Africa. Not because of the number of caps he has won, or his bank balance, or his police record. He is a success because of what he has overcome. Because success is like winning a boxing match. Everyone says congratulations but they forget how many times you've been punched in the face.

10

Frozen Solid

Roberto, twenty-nine years old
Cause of death: Ice
Cause of life: Old photos

'You are not dead until you are warm and dead.'

Those were the words that started one of the most memorable lectures I had in medical school, spoken by the renowned Home Office pathologist Dr Stephen Leadbeatter. Decades later, after travelling to the tinglingly beautiful mountains around Zermatt in Switzerland, I met a mountain medical rescue team who proved him to be right. They saved the life of Roberto after the world's longest cardiac arrest.

After a twenty-minute hike across ski fields, fluorescent trousers flashing past my eyes, I arrived at our meeting place. Iglu-Dorf is a frozen ice hotel tucked into the slopes on the Swiss side of the Matterhorn and where I first heard the story of a patient whose heart had stopped beating for nearly nine hours. I drank an 'Igloo coffee' to stay warm while I listened to the mountain medical rescue team's story, enjoying the Baileys liqueur that gave the drink an extra kick. But within a few sips, I developed a pounding headache, coming on too quickly to be the effects of the alcohol. Instead, the 3,135 metres I had ascended, 60 per cent of the altitude of Everest base camp, had started to affect my body. Despite the majestic surroundings, these cold wilderness regions where skiers and adventure seekers flock can quickly turn from a halo of beauty into a noose of danger. But along with peril, extreme cold can also bring hope for patients like Roberto, who had a cardiac arrest after freezing to death.

Roberto grew up in the bustling metropolis of Milan, staying in the city after university not for its fashion or food, but because of its proximity to the mountains. In just two hours, Roberto could leave his job as a chemist and be enveloped by the Italian Alps or Lombardy peaks. His love for these rugged heights was inherited from his parents, who would take the family on long hikes rather than lazy holidays on the beach. His mum worked as a specialist heart doctor, keeping her feet planted on the trails, but Roberto instead enjoyed being high in the air. He would ski over wild jumps, paraglide, ski and paraglide together at the same time. But Roberto found his true love at the age of twenty when he first tried climbing.

'Climbing is purified fun – all your problems in daily life just melt away. Even time somehow stops,' he told me.

Roberto and his friend Alessandro had long planned to tackle the 'Queen of the Dolomites', the highest mountain in the Dolomites region called Marmolada. The pair walked through the night, camped in the wilderness and began their ascent of a difficult, technical, vertical wall the next day. Roberto had planned to parasail from the top, but seeing unusually large amounts of blue ice hanging over ledges made him think twice. The weather was perfect as the friends made their first ascent. But as Roberto reached the first ledge on the South wall, unexpected storm clouds rolled over Marmolada. Alessandro took shelter against the rock in the pitch below, as Roberto recorded a video in which he says, 'You are not climbing in the Dolomites if it is not raining or snowing – but this is bad luck! Hail!'

Unknown to Alessandro as he sheltered, Roberto was trapped on the upper ledge, with freezing water and hail cascading down over the ice, on top of his body. For hours the storm raged, battering Roberto on the exposed face. Day turned to night before the weather broke. Alessandro climbed up to reach his friend, finding him lying unconscious on the craggy rock, his hands still gripping the brightly coloured rope. The whirl of a rescue helicopter got louder as Alessandro touched his friend. Roberto was frozen solid.

When tasked with a rescue on Marmolada, the helicopter emergency medical services of the Dolomites know their mission will be hard, bad and dangerous. A difficult mountain to climb, and even more difficult to rescue from. Their yellow helicopter rose from the sleepy village below to 2,800 metres, where Roberto was trapped. Soon after the rescue team reached Roberto, his heart stopped from this extreme cold – his body temperature was just 26C.

But even this doesn't beat the lowest temperature that a human has survived, a record still held by Anna Bågenholm, a Swedish radiologist. She had been skiing in Norway when she fell through a frozen stream, being trapped for over an hour. Her heart stopped for just over three hours with her temperature recorded as 13.7C. But although Anna was colder, Roberto's heart remained still for much, much longer.

'If someone had told me about a nine-hour cardiac arrest,' said Dr Alessandro Forti, who saved Roberto's life, 'I would never have believed it.'

Neither did Roberto's mum, a cardiologist who worked in the ICU for more than forty years. She used to tell Roberto a story about how she once needed to do CPR in the back of a speeding ambulance for nearly one hour – the patient died. Naturally, she had lost all hope of seeing her son alive again when told his heart had stopped for so long while the rescue helicopter was flying through a snowstorm. But survive he did, thanks to the very thing that killed him – the cold.

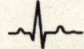

Some suggest a notable person who lived two lives may have done so with the help of hypothermia – Jesus. A paper published in the *Journal of the Royal College of Physicians of*

London called 'Resurrection or resuscitation?' describes how hypothermia induced by crucifixion may have simulated Jesus's death. His resurrection was actually resuscitation through gradual rewarming in a cave with a consistent temperature. Forget the divine intervention; it was more like divine insulation. Jesus was never dead because he wasn't warm and dead. So why does being cold help?

Imagine your brain as a bustling city, filled with office buildings, back streets, traffic, essential workers and a constant hum of activity. Every neurone, synapse and blood vessel are part of an elaborate, life-sustaining dance that happens even when you are sleeping. Now, picture a sudden blackout – instant chaos. All the lights go out, traffic signals go blank, trains halt, vital functions falter and the very infrastructure that keeps a city alive just stops. This is what happens during a cardiac arrest. As the heart stops, so too does the precious supply of blood and hence oxygen to the brain.

But what if we could slow down time in this moment of crisis? Get the city to go to sleep even before the blackout happens. Close the roads, stop the trains and empty the offices before the lights go off. Dramatically lowering the body's temperature offers just this chance – a means to protect the brain and vital organs by dialling down the body's metabolic demands before the blood supply cuts off.

Surgeons do this on purpose before replacing diseased main blood vessels that supply the brain. Deep hypothermic circulatory arrest is a medical technique used during complex cardiovascular surgeries including aortic arch repair, where temporarily stopping blood circulation is necessary. Patients are cooled to between 12C and 18C to reduce the metabolic demands of the brain and other vital organs. By significantly lowering the body's temperature, cellular metabolism slows, allowing organs to tolerate the lack of blood flow for a longer period without sustaining damage as the surgery continues.

The key point is that cooling must occur before any damage is done. In Roberto's case, his body gradually cooled down before his heart stopped. The cooling happened pre-emptively; the city went to sleep before the lights went out. It's tempting to think that cooling could help regardless of timing, but that's not the case. I assisted with clinical trials that aimed to replicate these benefits by cooling the body after someone had a cardiac arrest due to conditions like heart attacks. For years, doctors believed that hypothermia in these circumstances could protect the brain and improve survival rates. However, large clinical trials co-ordinated in the UK by my colleagues Jade Cole and Matt Wise showed that cooling at this later stage did not help. They found no significant differences in survival rates or neurological outcomes in patients who were cooled after a cardiac arrest compared to those who were not. By then, much of the brain damage had already occurred. Cooling people after the event couldn't reverse this damage, although avoiding high fevers during recovery may still prove beneficial.

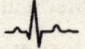

Frozen Solid

When the helicopter found Roberto freezing at just 26C, his heart had stopped due to the extreme cold. They winched him 30 metres off the sheer cliff face into the helicopter. With a long journey ahead through a snow-storm, the medics decided to use a special machine to do CPR on Roberto while flying at speed to safety. The device they used was a LUCAS (or Lund University Cardiac Assist System). It was invented by Norwegian paramedic Willy Vistung after he cared for a patient needing CPR in the back of an ambulance. Portable and battery-operated, the LUCAS and other similar devices deliver high-quality CPR while freeing up medical personnel to focus on other critical tasks in challenging environments.

After an hour of CPR, the helicopter landed at a nearby fifteenth-century regional trauma centre originally run by monks, as the weather conditions were too dangerous to travel further. While still having CPR from the LUCAS, Roberto was then driven by ambulance to the large Treviso hospital about 50 miles away. After nearly four and a half hours of CPR, doctors inserted the plastic pipes of an artificial heart/lung machine to restore blood flow to Roberto's organs. But like rugby player Rhys, Roberto still had no heartbeat. The team then very gradually rewarmed his body, 1 degree Celsius per hour, until finally eight hours and forty-two minutes after Roberto's cardiac arrest, they could restart his heart using a single electrical shock. It was the longest reported duration of CPR ever recorded. But records mean nothing unless a life is worth living and it would take weeks to find out.

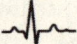

Intensive care is not actually about survival. It is not even about CPR or heartbeats or the binary outcomes of 'lived' and 'died'. Life isn't a spreadsheet. Of course, saving a life is a necessary first step, but giving life meaning once again is the journey I think about every day at work.

Medicine should not be about adding days to life, but about adding life to days. We aren't saving lives but resuscitating futures and hopes. I see every heartbeat we protect as a beat towards a meaningful, vibrant life beyond these walls where I spend so much time. Instead, the purpose of every intensive care admission is a discharge back to a life to be lived. I don't mend bodies but try to piece together the mosaic of someone's future, to breathe life back into the moments that make living worthwhile. Intensive care then is simply a bridge, not just spanning the gap between life and death, but leading to a path of restored purpose and joy. And this bridge is not a physical place or hospital wing. It's a village of people, a realm where we rebuild the story of someone's life, chapter by chapter.

Looking at my job this way helps me understand why so many patients yearn to return to the very places and activities that made them sick in the first place. Motorcyclists want to get back on the road, horse riders in the saddle, boxers want to fight again, runners to run. And climbers to climb.

Twenty-one days after freezing to death, Roberto was taken off his life support machine. His heart beat for itself, he breathed, opened his eyes and spoke. Yes, he had dressings on his chest where the thumping CPR machine had pressed down, keeping him alive for hours. And yes, he had dressings on his hands, where frostbite had damaged his skin and fingers. His right hand in particular was badly damaged, his muscles weak and Roberto had little control over his joints. But a journey back to his life had started.

The months of rehabilitation were tough. But Roberto stretched out his one hour per day at the hospital gym to three and then six and then eight hours a day. He was hyperfocused on his goal: to climb again. Roberto read about the story of Tommy Caldwell, a promising 23-year-old climber who suffered an accident that should have ended his career. While using a table saw during a home renovation in the Rocky Mountains of Colorado, he slipped and chopped off the index finger on his left hand above the knuckle. In his book, *The Push*, Caldwell details how he became the first person to complete a free ascent (climbing without ropes or equipment, using only your body) of Yosemite's El Capitan Dawn Wall through determination and resilience as he relearned how to climb after the accident, adapting his techniques to accommodate the loss of his finger.

Next, Roberto read about Jonathan Lessin, a retired physician whose efforts to mitigate his Parkinson's symptoms started a programme that would turn his climbing gym into a research facility. The improvement in Lessin's symptoms through climbing were so remarkable that his physical therapist put a newsletter in the Parkinson's clinic's waiting room. Before long, his climbing group of patients with Parkinson's had grown to over eighty participants before spreading to other gyms around the world.

After initial gains motivated by these new heroes Roberto read about, things seemed to slow down. His right hand remained stubbornly weak and he struggled to make sense of what had happened to him while unconscious in the intensive care unit. Time hung heavy; days passed slowly. Before Roberto could get better, before he could move onwards, he first needed to look back.

How many photos do you have on your phone? A thousand? Five thousand? Ten thousand? It may surprise you to check the true number. I have 18,500. If I looked at each of them for just a few seconds, it would take me over ten hours. And then there are the videos, the albums gathering dust under my bed, the stacks of old printed photographs still in their original holders. But don't worry – it's not just you and me.

Four and a half trillion photos have been stored on Google Photos, with 28 billion more uploaded each week. Social media users share 3.5 billion images every day. Look around at any event and the main activity seems to be taking bad, out-of-focus, digital copies of real-life experiences. My wife and I went to a concert by Kelly Jones, the singer-songwriter from the iconic Welsh band the Stereophonics. Held at a small venue, it was an amazing, intimate gig, but what radically transformed the experience was what wasn't there – any mobile phones. As we entered the 350-seat venue, our phones were sealed in individual opaque plastic bags for the duration of the performance. After the initial psychological discomfort this caused, the audience were transported to a place that is increasingly difficult to get to – the present moment. It was the greatest event I had ever been to partly due to the incredible orchestra, a faultless performance, but also because all 350 of us were truly there.

I realise this is an idealised version of life that doesn't factor in the utility of mobile phones. I don't pretend that I could give mine up for more than a few hours without a digital longing. We do have some family rules to help digital detoxification, including no phones in bedrooms and no work email allowed on personal devices. But there's a simple way to manage the neglected stories stored in the pixel past in our phones – look at your old photos. Don't wait until someone has died to look back. Don't print them out just for their funeral – look back now, look back every day.

When Roberto hit his low during rehabilitation, his friend Alessandro visited. Ever since waking from his coma, Roberto had no memory of the events that led to his cardiac arrest. There was a void where one of the most important experiences of his life should have been.

Although few of us have such a dramatic hole, as time passes your memory of events that played an important part in your own story will inevitably fade. And when there are gaps, these can easily be filled with myth, constructed memories or untruths. Missing memories are like lost pages in a book; they leave your story fragmented and make it harder to understand where you've been and where you're going. Like black holes in the galaxy of your mind, they can distort your path and pull you away from the direction of progress.

Roberto's father fixed this by playing the film Roberto had captured during that climb on Marmolada. After only a few frames, something very special happened.

'Bang – everything came back in one second!' Roberto said with a sense of joy on his face. 'Like a light was switched on. From that day, my recovery seemed to accelerate – to jump forward. I knew I would get back out to the mountains.'

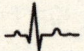

Looking back through your old photos, rather than just taking more and more, can be inspiring. The process can correct inaccurate memories and encourage comparison of our present with our past. Jo Hemmings, a leading UK behavioural psychologist, says, 'Taking the time to look back on our treasured memories can be truly beneficial for our well-being as it can help to evoke feelings of positivity and happiness. Because of this, and especially at times like this, we should take more time to appreciate and look back on them.'

Studies have shown that when people review the photos on their phones, it triggers not just positive emotions such as joy and love but it can strengthen our memory and even our relationships. These photos remind us of people, pets, places and activities that we love as well as helping us to remember the past. This has been shown to reduce our stress, enhance our mood and overall well-being. Looking back to reminisce on special moments creates an 'emotional bubble' where we return to the moment and manifest the feelings that were present. So too with the silly times in our lives, or even times we made mistakes. Laughing at embarrassing photos releases endorphins, our body's natural stress reliever. Seeing images of our friends and family in significant moments in our and their lives reduces cortisol and adrenaline, the hormones responsible for anxiety.

It is no wonder that we put photos in key places around our home. They act almost as potent drugs, altering perception and mood as we wander around our everyday life. Our mantelpieces, windowsills, shelves and sideboards, where many of us display our most treasured places and people in frames, have been shown to be the most peaceful places in our house. Research has also shown that having 'real' photos in our home provides regular positive psychological reinforcement by reminding us of social bond enhancement – essentially what and who are important to us.

So it is no wonder that just a few frames of the captured video helped Roberto remember. Photos can even help physical pain. In one study, participants were shown a series of twenty-six nostalgic images while hooked up to an fMRI machine and inflicted with varying amounts of pain using a heat generator attached to their wrist. The most sentimental photos massively reduced the pain experienced. Reminiscence stirred by images has a very powerful effect on many aspects of our mind, just like the photos of my Aunty Win at her funeral. I looked at them to remember, to reminisce, to bond and to help us get through the pain of tough times and of loss.

Yet, the ubiquity of photos on digital devices has led us to forget the value of looking at these images rather than only capturing them. In the 1970s, photographs were always the top item people would save from a house fire. Yet surveys done recently show that instead two thirds of people would first save their phone or computer. Less than one in ten people first grab photo albums from the flames; only one in a hundred choose original pieces of art.

The lessons here are clear. We should spend as much time looking back at old photos and videos as we spend taking them. Seeing people from the past may even motivate you to reconnect with those you had forgotten about or lost touch with. Why not have dinner with your old school friends? Pick up the phone and speak with that family member you fell out with for reasons you don't even remember or care about any more? Why not turn friends who accidentally morphed into strangers back into friends? This can all start from looking back at your pixel past, then saying hello once again.

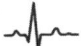

Three months and ten days after Roberto froze to death, he walked tall out of hospital. Moving into his parents' house at the foot of the Alps, he joined a new climbing gym. The first time Roberto cautiously placed his fingertips back on a rock face was a big moment.

'It was beautiful but not so beautiful,' he told me. 'I felt like a child climbing again, but I knew I would get better again and stronger with time.'

Happiness is not the absence of problems; it is having the ability to deal with them. A few months later, the Italian summer arrived; Aperol was everywhere. Roberto would normally be eagerly awaiting this time when the ice shelves melt and dry rock can again be gripped by his fingers, surrounded by groups of climbing friends, including Alessandro. But he was nervous. Lying on his bed as summer rays danced through a gap in his curtains, Roberto flicked through old photos and videos of him climbing in the mountains. A wide smile came across his face and his mum said, 'Just go, climb.' And so he did.

Six months after freezing to death, Roberto climbed again with Alessandro. The day before we spoke, Roberto had returned to the ice face nearest to his home, Monte

Bianco, and the next day he was meeting Alessandro at the Matterhorn where I drank my liqueur coffee.

'Aren't you scared?' I asked.

'You should never be scared of one bit of bad luck. Instead, I remember all the small bits of good fortune that added together to allow me to be here today, to allow my salvation.'

He showed me a photo on his phone of the helicopter rescue team, of his parents, of his friend Alessandro, of him lying frozen on the ground, of the face of Marmolada.

'Even if I were scared, my life is in the mountains. Don't be scared of your own life – it is the only one you have.'

11

A Funeral for my Friends

Matt, forty-four years old
Cause of death: TBC
Cause of life: A funeral

When I first told people at dinner parties that my next book was about death and funerals, their reaction was like a social experiment. Some people changed the subject faster than you can say 'eulogy', while others leaned in, morbidly fascinated, eager to discuss the inevitable with a touch of humour and grace. One stranger suggested I was trying to put the 'fun' in funerals. Nothing breaks the ice like the inevitable.

In writing this book, I've observed that the best in humanity often emerges in the darkest times. Funerals, while sombre, bring out stories of love, resilience and the indomitable human spirit. It's in these moments of collective grief that we see the true essence of community and compassion. We gather, we remember, and we find solace in shared memories, proving that even in the shadow of death, there is a light that binds us all.

I thought back to the last conversation I had with my Aunty Win, whose funeral started this book. I remember chatting in her house about a talk I was due to give to medical students about breaking bad news. I was pretty nervous about how to frame the talk, how to get over the importance of saving a death as well as a life in medicine. I wanted it to be positive despite the tough subject. Without much thought, she said to me, 'Well, sometimes darkness can show you the light.'

Looking back now at the slides for that talk, I included my Aunty Win's words on the final one. They accompanied an image taken in 1919, just five years after Win had been born. It is probably my favourite photograph of all time.

The photograph was taken by Sir Arthur Eddington on the remote West African island of Príncipe. Eddington tried to prove Einstein's theory of general relativity that mass bends light. Without our modern instruments, this could only be done using a simple black and white photograph during a very rare event – a total solar eclipse that passed directly over the island.

During a total solar eclipse, the Moon's disc passes in front of the Sun, obscuring its blindingly bright rays and allowing astronomers to study the dim light of background stars. By comparing photographs of these stars before and during the eclipse, Eddington could determine if the stars' positions had shifted due to the Sun's gravitational bending of space.

A Funeral for my Friends

The conditions on Príncipe when Eddington arrived were terrible. They were working under mosquito nets, with monkeys stealing their equipment. As the day of the eclipse arrived so too did an almighty rainstorm. Luckily, the clouds slowly cleared by midday, leaving just scattered mist as the eclipse started.

Eddington took sixteen photographic plates but only two contained enough stars to determine whether the light had been bent. The image I used to finish my talk was one of those photographs – starlight curving around the Sun, confirming that gravity did warp space-time. Einstein was right. The world changed.

This monumental discovery emerged from the darkness of the eclipse against the odds, against adversity. Perhaps what Aunty Win was trying to say was profound truths can only be revealed in shadow. Just as the stars' light bent around the Sun, sometimes in our own lives, moments of darkness can illuminate new paths and insights, showing us that even in the darkest times, we can find the light and the understanding we seek.

That is why I chose this topic. Not to be morbid, but because Aunty Win was right. Life consumes all that makes it precious – time, love and the lives of others. It can be dark, like war. I'm not sure any war can really be won. Everyone loses, just in different ways. Life is similar. But everyone wins, they just don't know it.

It was Charlie Chaplin who said, 'Life is a tragedy when seen in close-up, but a comedy in long-shot.' I take my job seriously, but I don't take myself too seriously. Perhaps we should do the same with life and with death. So why not put a little fun in funeral?

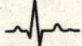

Of the main celebratory moments in life, it seems unfair not to experience or remember the two biggest – your birth and your funeral. And how many funerals have you been to where people say, 'I wish we didn't have to meet like this,' or you regret not having told the departed how much they had meant to you? What if you didn't need to meet like this and you could tell them? I couldn't go back to the start, my 0th birthday, so that just left my end . . .

Aunty Win's was the first funeral I had been to on my birthday. The second was my own. I hadn't died. But there I was, surrounded by friends, listening to what my mum, my dad, my wife and children really thought of me in their eulogy. My favourite song, 'Nightswimming' by R.E.M., was played by my good friend on his acoustic guitar.

The idea to hold my own funeral emerged during a whirlwind trip home from Australia. During the eight days I was staying with my parents, I gave a lecture, recorded my last audiobook, visited work colleagues, walked up a mountain, signed my will with the family solicitor and got drunk with my friends. It was the last two of these that resulted in this book.

As a completely healthy 44-year-old, my last wishes had lingered on my to-do list for years. After reading that forty-four was the average peak of happiness and well-being, it seemed there was a downhill gradient ahead. After one particularly difficult intensive care night shift months before in Australia, where another healthy 44-year-old had suddenly, unexpectedly met their maker, I couldn't sleep. Rather than wrestle with the sheets and remain trapped in my tumble dryer mind, I got out of bed in our rented house and wrote an email to our family solicitor in Wales. I asked if they could turn my ramblings into my last will and testament.

After the boring financial section came the part that really woke me up – what do you want for your funeral? After staring out of the window into the darkness, everything became clear, like a double espresso for my mind. I wanted a ceremony in the countryside, somewhere with mountains, green, a river, some birdsong. I'd love live music to be played – my favourite music. And home-cooked food. Definitely French wine for the guests, and good coffee. I hate bad coffee. Stretching my imaginary requests even further, I wrote, 'An outdoor log fire would be terrific.' In just ten minutes, I had fashioned my perfect day – one that I would never get to live.

A few days later, the bemused solicitor called. She had transformed my train-of-consciousness, post-night-shift ramble into equally confusing legal jargon.* But the document would need a wet signature. So this task was added

---

* 'In accordance with the Final Farewell Caffeine Statute, it is hereby mandated that only premium, high-quality, single origin, Arabica coffee ground with a conical burr shall be served at the funeral service.'

to my already crammed home visit schedule, wedged between a train ride back from London and meeting friends for a sunset beer.

A few months later, arriving late and flustered, I met my friends Ben and James at a rural pub overlooking the sea just before sunset. Fumbling through my backpack to find their token gifts (a koala pen and Tim Tams), two items fell to the ground. Tangled up in my headphones was my little red book that I carried everywhere to jot down notes and writing ideas. It landed on the ground open to a page on which was scribbled, 'Things that matter most . . . not things.' It had been what Cody had told me when we met in clinic after he had survived his cardiac arrest. I had been collecting the words and thoughts of people like Cody, who had seen both sides of life and death for years without knowing why. And next to my little red notebook was a copy of my will. When my friends asked what they were, I half-jokingly said, 'Oh nothing much, just the meaning of life and the best party that I will never be able to go to!'

I'm not sure who first suggested it and whether it was the jet lag or the beer, but by the time the Sun had set, the three of us had agreed to organise my living funeral. 'See you at my death!' were my parting words as I left the pub long after closing time.

I wasn't the first to spot the irony in the timing of a modern funeral. Between 1856 and 1906, organisations for the poor in Ireland paid for more than 25,000 people to move to the United States and Canada. In 1882, the government passed

A Funeral for my Friends

laws to help pay for the travel of more than 54,000 additional people. With this mass relocation was born the so-called American Wake. This was Ireland's heart-wrenching send-off for those crossing the ocean, where the only thing missing from the party was a corpse. It was a goodbye that felt like a funeral, except the guest of honour was very much alive. The goodbye bash was often as memorable as the life that had prompted it. But the Irish were not the first to this party.

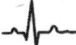

It was like I had been transported back to my first school disco – awkwardly hugging the walls before settling into an empty seat for solace. An unusual twist of fate had led me to one of the world's most prestigious theatres on London's South Bank. In my first year of medical school, I lived with eight other students, a jumbled crew that inexplicably meshed. Among them was Tim, an English literature student from the Welsh valleys who never let his stammer define him. Twenty-five years later, Tim, now an accomplished playwright, reached out to me unexpectedly.

'I've written a play about Aneurin Bevan – can you help with the medical details?' Tim asked in his email. I eagerly replied, 'Yes!' My theatre experience had been minimal since playing a non-speaking human-sized Christmas calendar at school, but I was thrilled at the opportunity. Two years on, I realised how closely linked theatre and medical practice truly are. We slice up the arts and sciences, as if they are different parts of a body. But really, they are just two eyes, looking at a slightly different view that is life. Both are needed to find your way around obstacles.

Every great theatrical production is anchored by a compelling story – one that intertwines human emotions, history, resilience and the quest for meaning. Tim's play, *Nye* – inspired by Bevan, the post-war health secretary and creator of the British NHS, and a fellow stammerer – captures these themes perfectly. Similarly, in my hospital, each patient carries a unique narrative. Even the rehearsal space sounded like echoes of the hospital – a blend of science, artistry and technical expertise, always grounded in the human experience. More purposeful engagement with the arts, be it theatre, music, poetry or dance, can be a transformative experience for us all. It certainly was for me. Serving as a medical adviser reignited my interest in public engagement by using movement, sounds and light rather than just my words. Drama can tell stories that go beyond mere facts, more real than non-fiction. Cross-disciplinary endeavours like this in your own life can enhance empathy, connections and open your mind. Of course there is a limit. You don't want to be so open-minded that your brain falls out. It is unfortunate that the fields of healthcare and theatre are facing funding cuts, diminishing their value and vision. Perhaps it is time to integrate more theatre into medicine and more recognition of the power of healing into theatre.

When Tim asked me to do this role as the medical adviser, I didn't realise that Michael Sheen would be playing the main character. I spent an hour chatting with the

Hollywood star at the coffee shop in the National Theatre. I told him about the plans for my living funeral and we connected over our shared experiences of loss. Michael told me how he would love to go back to Greek times not only to see the birth of theatre, but to quench his fascination with the Eleusinian Mysteries. Still starstruck and acting 'cool', I nodded along, pretending I knew what he was talking about. It turned out that the Greeks, and Michael Sheen, knew a lot more than me about living funerals.

Carved deep in the limestone entrance arch of the Monastery of Agios Pavlos in Mount Athens, Greece, are the words, 'If you die before you die you don't die when you do.' Picture these letters being scraped out a thousand years ago by hand in the then ancient city of Eleusis. This was a time and a place where secrets and mysteries held the power to transform those who dared to step into the inner sanctum. The Eleusinian Mysteries were a series of rituals and initiations shrouded in enigma, where participants grappled with the profound concept of death before they met their own demise. Much of it centred around the tale of Demeter and Persephone, a mother and daughter whose story outlines the cyclical nature of life, death and rebirth. Those who were lucky enough to be initiated into this clandestine world came to understand that death was not an end but a part of an eternal cycle.

The marble carving at Eleusis in Athens vividly depicts these sacred mysteries. At the centre of the relief, Demeter, the goddess of agriculture, offers a stalk of wheat to

A SECOND ACT

Triptolemus – the gift of food. Persephone, Demeter's daughter, stands beside them holding a fire torch, representing her journey between the underworld and the earth. It shows people playing instruments, making art, supporting others, drinking wine, bathing naked.

Fast forward to the 1990s, when Takiko Mizunoe became a trailblazer in Japan's entertainment industry. First, she shattered the glass ceiling of gender as a leading actress, then producer and director. But she also wanted to redefine the norms surrounding life's final curtain-call. This culminated in her decision to hold a living funeral on live television in 1992 as a healthy 78-year-old.

In this orchestrated farewell watched by millions, Mizunoe used the moment not as a morbid farewell but as a grand, heartfelt thank you note to the world. Mizunoe's parting message – 'to express appreciation to all those who have been dear to me while I am still alive' – wasn't just a farewell. She wanted a call to action to recognise the value of the present, the importance of expressing gratitude, and the profound effect our lives have on others. She lived another sixteen years and died at the age of ninety-four.

And so, although seemingly opposite, life and death are as close as 11 is to 1 on a clock face. This has been known and celebrated for thousands of years. So often, humans have thought of dying not as losing someone but discovering them. Yet we cannot discover ourselves through the modern accepted ceremony because we are already dead. Life changes behind you, when you turn around, when you stop looking. And sometimes we forget to turn around until it is all over. I wanted to turn around while I still could.

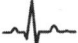

After flying back to Australia, I thought a lot about what we had agreed to do. I wondered if it would belittle those who are terminally ill, trivialise those who die before they should. I worried it may upset my family or be seen as an ego trip rather than a way to move beyond the self. And so I made a promise to myself that I would only have a living funeral if it were accompanied by a book to help others. My living funeral would be a way to get a little closer to the patients you have met in this book; people who have medically died before having a second chance at life – what I call a second act. I envisioned it as a book to help people learn valuable lessons from the patients I cared for who had faced death and then lived to tell their stories. Holding my funeral before I actually died allowed me a sneak preview of what matters while I still had time to do something about it.

My initial plan was to hold a service in my local village church in Wales, close to the pub where we had conceived the idea. But the vicar said they only provided funerals for 'Christians who had died' – two very reasonable basic requirements that I couldn't fulfil. It also felt narcissistic to centre the event just around me, especially given that friends of mine had terminal illnesses and their real funerals could come at any moment. So instead I took some advice from writer Helen Keller, the first deaf and blind person to earn a college degree, who said, 'I would rather walk with a friend in the dark, than alone in the light.' So instead I would organise a group event with my friends so we could walk towards the dark together.

Christmas that year soon passed in a blaze of ill-fitting gifts and as the January blues hit many at home, I baked in the Western Australian sun. Weeks had turned to months since the idea had been agreed and finding a mutually convenient date was tricky. I wondered if we would ever really go through with the scheme.

Then, in that weird post-Christmas television period just after New Year, I flicked on to the 1986 cult classic film *Ferris Bueller's Day Off*. During the opening sequence, after Ferris convinces his parents that he is too sick to go to school, he says a line repeated during the last reflective moment in the final scene. 'Life moves pretty fast. If you don't stop and look around once in a while, you could miss it.'

Hearing that for the second time made me physically stand up from the sofa and send a message to my friends. The only date most people had been able to make was very inconvenient for me. But hearing that movie line made me think, 'So what!' *Vitam vive*.

My message read:

A Funeral for my Friends

Strange request alert!

To help me write a book, I am planning a 'living funeral' for a group of friends. You would need to choose:

- A song
- A course for a meal or a drink
- A reading that could be anything from a poem to a long joke

I have organised an independent celebrant to conduct the event where we take it in turn to read out each other's choices below and a eulogy written by the people who love you.

The transport is pretty tight, so please only bring one small bag and there is a no-phones policy so we can only argue with each other rather than random strangers on the internet.

I've found a remote mountain cottage with a hot tub and a view of some green mountains. I'll pay for all accommodation/food/drink/car hire because spending time with friends matters. Then a year later I'll be visiting home from Australia again and it would be great to catch-up to see how your lives may have changed from the experience . . .

Oh, and the only date we can all do is 25 January – my birthday. I had originally thought this would be a problem. But thinking about it more, what better day is there to have my own funeral?

Can you come??

Love Matt x

A SECOND ACT

I invited a varied group of friends who had all had different experiences of loss in their lives. Old friends from school, new dads I met at the school gate, strangers I first met over the dissection table at medical school who, through the extraordinary highs and lows at the coalface of medicine, I am bonded to for ever.

Those with the most personal connection with death were perhaps the most engaged with the experiences and also seemingly the most adapted. Even the happiest. Humans are remarkable at adapting to the situations in which they can be thrust. I wondered how difficult experiences may have impacted on the personalities of my friends gathered around me.

Humans are notoriously poor at predicting what will make them happy, a phenomenon known as affective forecasting. This is especially true when it comes to money. For instance, a shorter commute can make you as happy as a 40 per cent pay rise, a paid holiday from your boss can be more satisfying than receiving cash, and having more free time often brings greater happiness than having more money. Yet people frequently assume that more money is the key to happiness. We also adapt to radical change. The lottery win will make you happier for a period and the accident sadder for a period. But we often regress to a norm. Humans are remarkably resilient.

But should I have travelled to my funeral with my family, my wife, my children and not my friends?

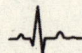

A Funeral for my Friends

The poet Meghan O'Rourke in her book *The Long Goodbye*, written in the wake of her mum's death, said, 'The friends we most love do become a physical part of us, ingrained in our synapses, in the pathways where memories are created.'

She was right. Your friends are a part of you, you of them. And friendships reshape our brain and body in profound ways. Neuroscientist David Eagleman explains how people we love become a part of us physically: 'People you love become part of you — not just metaphorically, but physically. Your brain refashions itself around the expectation of their presence.'

While the idea that we become the average of the five people we spend the most time with may be overly simplistic, this underscores the profound influence that social bonds have on our neurological framework, on our life. Our brains change their neuronal pathways around the expectation of good friends being in our lives.

Psychological studies consistently show that stable, healthy friendships are crucial for our well-being and longevity. Individuals with strong social networks are more satisfied with their lives and less likely to suffer from depression. They also have a lower risk of dying from heart problems and chronic diseases. A landmark study of more than 300,000 people found that poor social connections increase the risk of premature death more than smoking twenty cigarettes a day. Time to put down the lighter and pick up the phone.

Friendships offer more than just emotional support. They

have tangible effects on our physical health. Lydia Denworth, author of a book on the science of friendship, highlights how social isolation affects the immune system, leading to increased inflammation and a weakened immune response. Friendships change our white blood cells. Conversely, socially integrated individuals tend to have lower blood pressure, better sleep quality and faster healing times. Strained friendships, on the other hand, are significant predictors of chronic illness.

The impact of friendships on our response to stress is particularly noteworthy. Studies reveal that blood pressure and heart rate reactivity are lower when individuals face stressful tasks with a supportive friend by their side. In one fascinating experiment, participants even perceived a hill as less steep when accompanied by a friend, underscoring the psychological and physical comfort that friendships provide.

But loneliness isn't just an issue for older people. This protective effect of friendships extends across all age groups and while health interventions targeting loneliness often focus on older adults, younger individuals can also benefit. If life were a three-legged stool, we often let it lean to one side and become unstable. We focus our time on work and family, neglecting the third leg: ourselves. Yet spending time with good friends is likely to be more beneficial than any medication I could prescribe.

While books on rekindling romantic relationships are stuffed on to the shelves in the self-help section of libraries and bookshops, the quiet power of friendships deserves equal recognition, if not more. As we navigate life's challenges, the support and presence of friends without benefits offer even more advantages than those with their clothes off.

To make the most from the retreat, I wanted to capture not only the plans I had made in my will but also the lessons I had been collecting from patients in my little red book. Flicking through the pages, I wrote down the lessons scribbled in different colour pens from patients who would make up this chapter.

From Chapter 7, Alex showed us that life is driven by chance, so I didn't want to over-plan. But I did want us to overcome the spotlight effect, worrying about what others thought of us, by doing the weird things in life. Although there were just eight of us there, we also wanted to remember and name the dead who couldn't join us.

Luca in Chapter 2 told us words have power, as do green spaces in nature. Our experience would include messages from those close to us, words from history, and that we should be surrounded by the great, green outdoors.

Cody's meaning in Red Dust, Chapter 3, was found through moments, not physical things. I wanted to minimise the number of personal items people brought, especially those that distract rather than connect. Instead, we would focus on a few meaningful activities needing us to work together.

Summer helped us choose the right people to be surrounded by. We all have friends who are perfect for some occasions yet terrible for others. She also reminded us how life can change dramatically from just a single event. I hoped our funeral would be the start of a change, not the end. I also brought along three of my favourite games that we had never played together as a group of friends after thinking about how Tetris has transformed Summer's life. Pass the Pigs is a silly game of rolling miniature rubber pigs for points perfect for the airport, while the magnet game Kluster was played as a drinking game over lunch, leaving Werewolf for the second sober evening after allegiances had formed, secrets exchanged and thoughtful espionage was needed.

After Mike drowned in Chapter 5, he realised that together we are stronger. Collaboration and shared efforts are crucial for survival with life's greatest achievements coming from collective effort. So I would ask each of my friends to bring along a particular skill to the trip.

Jen's heart taught us to enjoy what you have now, rather than waiting for that perfect time to come. There is never a good time for eight people with busy lives and demanding jobs to meet. But we would need to just go with one date even if it were not ideal. To *Vitam vive* – live life.

When Alex survived his severe allergy, he found that music was the operating system for his soul. He started to engage in activities he enjoyed despite not being great at them. Music was essential for the trip, and I had the perfect idea.

Kai's change in pace led to his second act through more quit, less grit. We all need to live a life worth remembering so a memento would be needed to stop our funeral from quickly fading into the background clamour of life. And our experience may even lead to someone giving up what is not right for them. Rhys told us to leave our demons behind. This was the perfect space between the stimulus of busy lives to find the responses we want in our future selves, not the versions of us that we ruminate on at night. And finally, Roberto swept off the digital dust settled on old images, uncovering memories that should be reignited. I would travel with a clutch of old photos, keys to unlock good times and good people, passed but not to be forgotten.

Armed with this list of demands, I felt like a new breed of travel agent for the end of days. I typed 'Rural cottage/green mountain/French wine/log fire/sleeps eight' into my web browser and an idyllic cottage nestled in the French Pyrenees quickly flashed up. It even had a wood-fired hot tub with a strict 'no clothes' policy that could help us loosen our inhibitions. With the accommodation found, good home-cooked food was outsourced to my Sicilian *amico*, and my oldest school friend was the perfect choice for the live music, being a talented singer and guitarist. Other roles were constructed – someone to capture the event through a painting, and another as official photographer. We had a French speaker book a local restaurant with not a single review, leaving its quality entirely to chance, and the party animal would source the wine.

To make the experience more authentic, I asked a French-based British celebrant called Mark to conduct the service. Having worked as a teacher before running a café, Mark changed his own lifestyle radically a few years previously, moving to a remote part of France to set up his own business. He understood the power of reflection, was intrigued by the idea of a living funeral and agreed to help, on a few conditions. To make it an authentic experience, Mark wanted to speak with our families so he could write a fitting eulogy for each of us. We each needed to choose a reading, be it a poem or a short passage, that meant something to us. Everything, including the song we had each chosen to be played, needed to be kept secret until the big day. It perfectly matched the themes from my will and the messages from people's second acts.

Asking your partner, mum, dad, brother or sister to write your eulogy is hard. It is fair to say that the reactions were very mixed. While I overheard my wife and daughters laughing with Mark as they retold notable events from my life, for others this wasn't so. Simply imagining someone you love not being there was too difficult for some. They couldn't do it, no matter how fictional the funeral. For others, it caused conflict and disagreement. Despite being the most certain thing in life, death is still too much for many to contemplate.

Of course, a living funeral is really just theatre. We weren't really going to die. But neither did the people in this book. Their hearts did stop for minutes or hours, but death is not that. If it were, we would all die more than 100,000 times per day between the normal beats of our hearts. But perhaps we should consider each of the tiny pauses as a chance to live again; something more powerful than even death.

But even theatre can be profoundly moving. We knew

we weren't really dead, and we knew that tomorrow would come. Yet this dress rehearsal truly mattered. In fact, the use of candlelight and reminiscing about the past might actually mirror what happens just before the final curtain-call in our lives.

The day

I soon received enthusiastic yet bemused replies from seven close friends made during different phases of my life, all willing to take on this experiment. With flights booked, songs chosen and eulogies written, we were ready to travel to a place we had never been before – geographically or spiritually.

Touching down at Toulouse airport, spirits were high for all of us. The two-hour drive into the mountains was stretched out to over five as French farmers protested against government reforms by digging up sections of the motorway. By nightfall, the eight-seat hire car that had presumably been designed for jockeys started to make the afterlife appealing. We counted down the miles one by one. Eventually, arriving to French onion soup homemade by Tom, who had arrived earlier in the day, a roaring fire and the promise of a special weekend was reward enough. The next day we had an amazing long lunch at the local restaurant that we took a chance on even if the vegetarian soup did come complete with a floating carcass from an unidentifiable mammal. We passed around old photos, each like a bookmark to shared pages, bringing long-forgotten moments back to life and rekindling emotions that have lingered in the background.

We arrived back at the cottage as the setting sun was framed by a mountain glacier on the right and lush green trees on the left. Ben took some amazing photos as good coffee was brewed, wine poured and homemade gnocchi, cooked the traditional Sicilian way by my Italian-speaking friend Corrado teaching native Welsh speaker Dave. The log fire burned under an outdoor hot tub that was gaining heat for later that night. There were no mobile phones to vibrate, no television showing tragic news that would distress but not directly affect us. We all wore scruffy jeans, T-shirts and had ruffled up hair apart from Corrado. Instead, he wore an old, long nightshirt gown, sown by an elderly lady for his best friend Paolo, a Capuchin monk living in Jerusalem. To complete the integration of cultures, Corrado took a leaf from my best man Jon's Scottish heritage by forgetting to pack spare underwear, hence taking an oath not of celibacy but of commando contemplation. The spotlight effect clearly had never arrived in Sicily.

It was everything I had hoped for. This was our church. We spoke about the people who couldn't be there, saying their names including friends, parents, brothers and sisters who had died. Soon a serious hush fell over our group. Mark the celebrant stepped outside, where we were gathered. We put down our glasses, took a deep breath and listened.

I have great pleasure to formally declare you all dead. That's it. It's all over. You can't see any of your loved ones again. You can't achieve anything again. You can't touch, feel, smell, emote again. You are a blackness. You've gone. You do not exist. You're dead. Your time is up. Your legacy begins.

What is your legacy? What and who have you left behind? How do you feel about your life so far? How do you feel about what you have done and said on this planet in the short time you have had here?

Because today is your funeral. Today is the day your loved ones unite in grief to say goodbye to you. What does it mean to hear the words of your loved ones in your eulogies? What does it mean to experience dying today? What does it mean to hear that today is the funeral of Matthew Philip Govier Morgan?'

What followed was hard to describe. Each of us in turn had a candle lit, we died, we listened to the words put together by those who love us, read aloud by friends old and new. We each had a reading, then our chosen song was played beautifully by Carlo. Dave served the Italian food he had been taught to make by Corrado. James painted the scene despite not being a painter. Ben captured moments using his camera, while Jon opened the wine and Tom tended the fire. There was great laughter and deep joy. And there were tears. Eight grown men, silent, listening, crying. An antidote to toxic masculinity. Much that was said was tough to hear, tough to say.

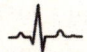

Life has a way of carving its stories into your face, hidden in expressions that only come out now and then. Each of us in our own time had faced moments that tested our resolve, that demanded more from us than we thought we could give. We have all known the sting of hardship, the weight of burdens seemingly too heavy to bear. Yet this was how we got here, how we were forged. Sometimes you don't need clouds to have silver linings.

We had all felt loneliness and the pang of despair. And the scars we hide are not symbols of suffering, but emblems of resilience. Yet we keep them under wraps. We are all cracked, but not broken. Because in these shared struggles there is a silent camaraderie, a recognition that we are all bound by the threads of our trials. We've known the sleepless nights, the heart-wrenching decisions, the quiet moments of doubt. Quiet people often have the loudest minds. We've felt the suffocating pressure of expectations and the crushing weight of disappointment. And yet, despite it all, we have found ways to rise, to adapt, to continue moving forward.

I say this because our tough times as a group are not unique or even that bad when compared with the weight of the world. They are instead common ground upon which we all stand, today or tomorrow or yesterday. They remind us that while our journeys may differ, the essence of our struggles is universal. It defines our humanity.

I watched the sequence of crying take an interesting path. It was often not the person whose turn it was to die

A Funeral for my Friends

that would cry. It was instead their friends, hearing about the life of others and feeling what their loss would mean. My oldest friend Carlo, a logical maths-loving actuary geek and an amazing guitarist, struggled to play what should have been an easy song for him as I died. Jon, a GP who listened to tales of sadness daily in his clinic, had a tear in his eye as Corrado died, whom he had only just met. And even if it were the dying person who cried, it was not their own demise that got to them – but hearing the words written by their parents, their kids, their wives, their friends.

All men cry, but they do it alone, or drunk. We were together and almost sober. A lot of men struggle to open up to anyone, let alone other men. Our culture beats into us the understanding that 'being a man' means not showing any vulnerability. We fear being judged as feeble by other men, unattractive by those we desire, and unfit by society. It's this fear that drives some men to ridicule one another when these emotions surface. But I didn't cry because I was sad, or weak, but because I was grateful. Grateful that we get a second shot at life. Every day. Grateful that I can try again and again to reconcile the passions and the rage that is a life. But I didn't expect how transformational this day would be.

We had done everything on the list, followed the advice of all the patients you have read about. We looked a lot like that marble carving of the Eleusinian Mysteries that Michael Sheen had told me about, although I'm not sure even the Greeks could fit eight men naked and crying into a hot tub. It was like the best ever birthday, with priceless gifts of words and time. After the crying had stopped, the gnocchi eaten and the songs had ended, Mark the celebrant stood up and licked his finger. One by one, he touched the flames of each of our candles that were lit as we died. As he did, he said:

> As I extinguish these candles, I am pleased to announce that you are no longer dead. You are fully alive, ready to embrace the rest of your life to the fullest.
>
> May you all recognise the profound impact your life has on those around you.
>
> May you all cherish your loved ones and understand how your existence enriches theirs.
>
> May you all be blessed with good health, joy and love, experiencing a long life filled with happiness.
>
> And even when you face challenges with your health, experience less joy, or endure the loss of loved ones, remember life isn't easy, but it's the only one you've got.

In one hundred years, you will be dead. Someone else will live in the home you worked so hard to build. Someone else will own all of your things. Your car will be scrap metal, your wedding ring on someone else's finger you have never met. Your descendants will hardly know who you were. You may be a portrait on a wall but your history, your photos and videos will be digital dust. You won't even be in anyone's memories.

A Funeral for my Friends

And I say this not in the name of nihilism nor despair. I say this to scream at you for hope and freedom. Read this again and then think about the 95 per cent of things that you have worried about this week. They don't matter.

Nothing is really yours. Nothing truly belongs to you. You borrow time, people, memories and joy, much like books from a library. Some pages will be stained with tears, others with coffee, and some might go missing. But your story will eventually end, your book will return to the shelf, and someone else will borrow it.

So make this book transform your story. Let it change your life now by listening to the whispers of those who have lived a second act. You don't need to die to experience this transformation. Why not turn your 'life 1.0' into 'life 2.0' now?

Life gets easier once you realise life's not getting any easier. If this is rock bottom, at least it is solid ground. The world is so beautiful and life so short. Don't let your life be wasted on living; don't let your funeral be wasted on your death.

'I began to think that, you know, in reality, we often say that I hope to go to heaven when we die. In reality, we go to heaven when we're born.'

— *Astronaut James Lovell*

Epilogue

'Life should not be a journey to the grave with the intention of arriving safely in a pretty and well-preserved body, but rather to skid in broadside in a cloud of smoke, thoroughly used up, totally worn out, and loudly proclaiming "Wow! What a Ride!"'

Hunter S. Thompson

Our living funeral was the ultimate reality check. It nudged us not to wait for that special occasion to celebrate the people who matter. In ICU, the hours are long, but the years are short. The same is true in life. Too often the admin of existence gets in the way of living. What you mean to say is not said, what you say is not heard, what is heard is not understood and what is understood is not done. Instead, our funeral forced us not to 'be' things, but to do things. Like in life, none of us really knew what to expect from the experience or knew what we were really doing there.

But in the end, it was like attending the premiere of our

own life's movie, reminding us all to make each scene count and appreciate unexpected plot changes. The ultimate twist was being able to see the tears, the laughter and the love. But it was also an opportunity to read our reviews while we could still make edits, and fix any plot holes.

But at the end of the trip, as I packed away my toothbrush and made emergency repairs to the hot tub not used to housing eight men, I wondered, *would anything really change?*

Six months later I found out. As compressed winter nights turned into long summer-stretched evenings, I caught up with my friends during another trip home from Australia. While waiting at the airport, I received an email requesting a reference for Tom. He had started volunteering with underprivileged kids in London, giving them a role model to aspire to, promising that better things could lie ahead. Then I found out that James had quit his job, swapping a long commute for a role closer to home for less money, but more time. Our Italian *amico* Corrado had just returned from a cycling trip abroad, finally carving out time for himself alongside being a great husband and dad to a big family. Dave, a busy GP, had thrown himself into organising a community festival in Devon, filled with music, good food and raising money for a local charity. Jon ended years of planning a big trip to Japan by booking flights during his lunch break, resulting in a magnificent few weeks spent there with his family. Carlo abandoned his long-sought early retirement plans, pulling money out of his theoretical actuarial spreadsheet and instead jointly buying land in

Spain with his sister. And I chatted about all of these life changes with Ben, as we played cricket for a local team, bowling our first balls for more than twenty-five years. We were terrible, and we didn't care. Life should be a verb, a doing word; not a noun, just a name. But the changes we felt after our funeral weren't always about making grand, sweeping decisions. Instead, the trip was a constant reminder to put things in perspective. When we had a shitty day, reflecting on that experience helped us all reset and approach situations with a clearer mind. To widen the gap between stimulus and response.

But what about me? I had spent the last year meeting cardiac arrest survivors, trying to see life through a different lens, where the mundane becomes meaningful. I had moved my family across the world to find a better life, new meaning. But my living funeral had changed me too.

The advantage of it pissing down in Wales for half of the year is that the grass here really is greener. Absence doesn't just make the heart grow fonder but can remind us that the heart was there in the first place. It can be hard to see what is in front of us sometimes.

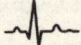

On a brisk January morning in 2007, amid the bustle of a Washington metro station, a man lifted a violin above the sounds to play Bach. After five minutes, just one middle-aged man noticed the music, pausing for just a beat before walking on. A minute later, the violinist's hat felt the first

Epilogue

dollar hit, tossed by a woman without stopping to see it land. Six minutes in, a young man leaned against a wall for a moment. Ten minutes into the performance, a toddler halted, spellbound, only to be tugged away by his mother. After forty-five minutes, 2,000 commuters wrapped up in their morning routines had blurred past him, only six people had stopped to listen, and around twenty added money to the hat without a pause. This totalled $32.

The violinist was Joshua Bell – one of the world's most acclaimed musicians. Just two days earlier, he had filled a Boston theatre, where fans paid $100 each to hear him play the very same pieces echoing around that metro station.

Do you recognise beauty? Do you pause to cherish it? If we cannot spare a moment to appreciate one of the finest musicians in the world, at the peak of his craft, using the finest instrument, what else might you be missing as life hurries by?

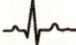

I was sitting next to a deep crystal blue river on a sunny day in Australia a few weeks before my flight to catch-up with my friends when I knew we were going home for good. My wife's dad had just been diagnosed with dementia and I went for a walk around the local village where I found *The Alchemist* by Paulo Coelho at a book exchange. I read it in a single sitting that afternoon as pins and needles ran over my legs from sitting still for too long on the river's edge.

The novel describes the journey of a young Andalusian shepherd named Santiago. Feeling bored by his pastoral life, he decides to pursue his recurring dream of finding treasure in the Egyptian pyramids. As Santiago travels, he meets characters who make him realise that the treasure he seeks is not the material wealth but rather spiritual enlightenment and self-knowledge. The climax of the quest is when Santiago finds the treasure right back where he started, at home in Spain. This revelation completes a full circle, emphasising that we are all in the pursuit of distant dreams and desires and can overlook the riches that were always present at the beginning. True fulfilment and happiness often lie within and where we least expect them. This isn't just a cliched meme. It has real-world implications for your own life even if you are just walking along the road next to your house. It had taken this journey through the lives and deaths of others, and then the life and imagined death of me, to realise what had been there all along.

So why did we decide to pack up our home once again after moving? Why organise another leaving party? Why leave a place where most 'things' are better?

We came home because writing this book had taught me so much. Life isn't about things — it's about people and belonging. We missed our family, our friends, our colleagues, our home. We missed the thing that my fellow Australian Cody wanted so badly: meaning. We have no regrets about having left. I learned so many new skills and ways of working, made friends through new colleagues, travelled to

Epilogue

new places. Equally, we have no regrets about coming home to our parents, our dog, our people and our sense of belonging. Our meaning. It can be described using an old Welsh word *Cynefin* – the place where we feel we belong to the people and landscape, the sights and sounds. I think of it in a different way. Yes, 'home' can sometimes be shit. But it is my shit.

And we don't regret it when it is shit. And even if we did, it is better to choose your regrets rather than have them placed upon you. Staying positive doesn't mean you have to be happy all the time. It means that even on hard days, you know there are better days to come. Sometimes you need to shake that snow globe, so the snow is falling all around. Even though it is hard to see through, it is exciting. And the snow will settle. The air will clear.

What is more, the meaning that so many find elusive doesn't have to be so grand as a move to the other side of the world or a change of job. It can be small, temporary. It can be volunteering alongside your job before taking that big move like my friend Tom. It can be to pick up that musical instrument once again that you haven't played for twenty years like Alex. It can be closer to home than you think. Meaning it can be small. But just enough to bring your life back to life.

When you were born, you had 300 bones. Now you have only 206. Those ninety-four bones have not disappeared – they have fused together. Life can sometimes feel like a loss or constant change. But losing things can sometimes make you stronger. Life fuses you together. And finding meaning also doesn't have to be a shiny new thing. The nearest exit is often behind you, and so going back to some place or some phase of your life is not a backwards step. Sometimes this can be hard to see. But remember, you can't even see your own eyes. You already know many of the lessons in this book, but it important who is telling them to you. It can take a lifetime to take your own advice. Don't live an unlived life. Because there is no such thing as an after-life crisis.

I ended my first book, *Critical*, with some simple words of advice: 'Work hard, ask questions, be kind.' If I were to rewrite that book today, it would instead read, 'Be kind, listen for the answers, work hard at living life.' I now realise that like working in ICU, the whole of your life is an emergency. Every second counts. Myriad books offer advice on living a better life, with insights from business leaders to spiritual gurus. They all share a common perspective: that of the living. But the dead can teach us much more. I think we all should have a funeral before we die.

Acknowledgements

Thank you to Charlotte Seymour, my wonderful literary agent at Johnson and Alcock, who took a chance on an unpublished stranger over five years, and now three books, ago. Thank you to my fantastic editor, Frances Jessop, who untangled my ideas and weaved them into something so much better. David Edwards has been an amazing copy-editor – if this book makes sense, it's entirely their fault. Thanks to the whole team at Simon & Schuster.

Thank you to my mum and dad for their unwavering support, encouragement, cutting the grass and saying, 'Same rules apply.' Thank you to my wife, Alison, and my two daughters, Evie and Mimi, for giving me the greatest reasons for coming home after a hard day's work in critical care.

Thanks to Jake for his wonderful photos and all my friends who agreed to come to their own funeral.

To my wonderful colleagues at the University Hospital of Wales, BMJ, the Royal Perth Hospital, Curtin University and Cardiff University – thank you for your hard work, support and care. Thanks to BMJ group for publishing my columns, allowing me to use them as inspiration and to Dr Peter Brindley, who has been a hugely important writing companion for years. Thanks to the software team at Ulysses, whose software was used to write all the words in this book. Thanks to Rhian and the team at 2Wish for their essential work.

Thanks to Dale Gardiner, the national Clinical Lead for Organ Donation in the UK, for putting me in touch with Jen. Thanks to Jerry Nolan and the Resuscitation Council (UK) for helping with the CPR section. Thanks to Mark Rind, the independent celebrant who lives in France, for conducting such an amazing service. Thanks to Andrew Billen for his support over the years and Lyndy Cooke at Hand Held Events. Thanks to Paul Bloom and Kenneth Cukier, who I met at the wonderful HowTheLightGetsIn Festival, as well as David Cain, who gave me the idea about writing a letter to yourself. Thanks to Professor Matt Wise, who introduced me to patients having a cardiac arrest through his world-leading research trials, and to Thomas Keeble for his work supporting them. Thanks to my cousin Dr Claire Williams for getting in touch with those we have cared for together in the past. Thanks to Luigi Camporota, Antony Garvey, Crawford Deane, John Chatterjee, Alessandro Forti, Anders Santoft, Giacomo Strapazzon, Ed Litton and Robert Larbalestier.

This book has been written in countless cities, countries and time zones. It has been fuelled by a never-ending stream

Acknowledgements

of coffees and pains aux raisins. Two places deserve a special mention – the Coco Belle Espresso Bar in Perth, which made the best banana bread, and the Sully Inn for their Guinness. Thanks to Joni Mitchell, Cigarettes After Sex and Noah Kahan for their music that has been playing on loop.

But most of all, thank you to everyone in this book who has given me their stories, their words and their trust. Thanks to the patients who lived who I shall remember for a very long time, and to those patients who died who I shall remember for ever.

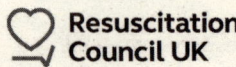

Resuscitation Council UK

Your actions could save a life.

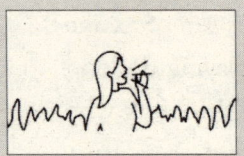

A cardiac arrest is when someone's heart suddenly stops beating, and their breathing is abnormal or has stopped.

Without quick action, the person will die.

Check for danger, then immediately follow these simple steps to give the person their best chance of survival:

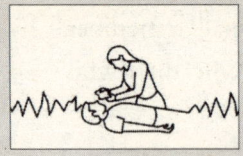

1. Shout for help.
   - Shake them gently.

2. Look and listen for signs of normal breathing.
   - Look for the rise and fall of their chest.

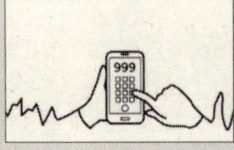

3. Call 999. Put the phone on loudspeaker and tell them you are with someone who is not breathing.

4. Start chest compressions.
   - interlock your fingers
   - place your hands in the centre of the chest
   - push down hard and then release twice per second, and don't stop.

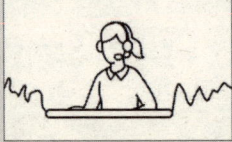

The ambulance call handler will help you.

5. The ambulance call handler will tell you where the nearest automated external defibrillator (AED) is. If someone is with you, ask them to fetch it and bring it back.

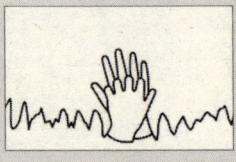

Do not leave the person if you are on your own.

6. If you have a defibrillator, switch it on and follow the instructions. It will tell you exactly what to do.

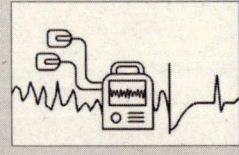

7. Continue CPR until:
   - the AED asks you to pause while it reanalyses and gives another shock if needed
   - a paramedic arrives and tells you what to do
   - the person shows signs of life.

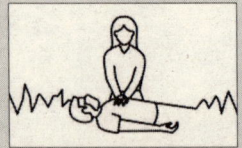